Keeping Your Child Healthy with Chinese Medicine

A Parent's Guide to the Care and Prevention of Common Childhood Diseases

Bob Flaws

BLUE POPPY PRESS

Published by:

Blue Poppy Press
A Division of Blue Poppy Enterprises, Inc.
3450 Penrose Place, Suite 110
Boulder, CO 80301
(303) 447-8372

First Edition July, 1996
Second Printing March, 1999

ISBN 0-936185-71-6
Library of congress Catalog Card #96-94842

COMP Designation: Original work using a standard translational terminology

Printed at Johnson Printing
Cover design by Jeff Fuller, Crescent Moon

10, 9, 8, 7, 6, 5, 4, 3, 2

Preface

This book is a layperson's primer on children's diseases according to Traditional Chinese Medicine. It is intended primarily for parents. It is not a clinical manual for professional practitioners. Rather, it contains what I regard as the most important information for parents on how to keep their children healthy and well. It includes a number of home remedies and describes to parents the kinds of treatments professional practitioners of Chinese medicine are likely to recommend for various children's diseases. The diseases covered are loosely arranged longitudinally. That means that they appear in a rough chronological order corresponding to when in the child's development that disease or condition is likely to crop up. Thus this list begins with neonatal jaundice and colic. Although the list ends with various epidemic and infectious diseases, such as measles and mumps, the reader should know that these may strike at any age. The last category of complaints are traumatic injuries which may also occur at any age but tend to occur more after the child is playing outside with other children.

If your child becomes ill and simple home remedies do not result in obvious and timely improvement, my best advice is to see a professional practitioner of Chinese medicine trained in pediatrics. If your child needs to see a Western MD, any responsible professional practitioner of Chinese medicine will make that referral when truly necessary.

Chinese medicine is a rising star in Western health care today. It provides great insight into many health problems not dealt with completely or satisfactorily by modern Western medicine. In particular, Chinese medicine provides simple to understand reasons for why we get sick the way we do and, based on those reasons, tells us what we ourselves can do both to prevent and treat those diseases. Thus Chinese medicine is an enlightening and empowering medicine, returning a great deal of autonomy and the responsibility that goes with that autonomy back to the individual.

As a clinician, my day to day work mainly focuses on the treatment of diseases which have already occurred. However, it is an ancient and long-standing principle in Chinese medicine that the superior doctor teaches patients how to prevent disease rather than just treating diseases which have already arisen. Treating disease after it has developed is likened in the Chinese medical classics to digging a well after one has become thirsty or forging spears after war has been declared. Therefore, I have a great desire to share the preventive and self-treatment wisdom of Chinese medicine with as large an audience as possible, and this and other books I have written for lay readers are an outgrowth of that desire.

The material in this book is derived from three main sources. First is my training in Chinese medical pediatrics I received at the Shanghai College of Traditional Chinese Medicine. Second is the Chinese medical literature on pediatrics. And third is my own clinical experience as a professional practitioner of acupuncture and Chinese medicine over the last 18 years. But just as importantly, as a parent myself, I and my wife have been called on to make many of the hard choices discussed in this book. Like you parents who are reading this book, I too have lost many nights of sleep staying up with a sick child. Thus much of the information in this book comes not just from my experience of treating other peoples' kids but from applying this knowledge within the proving ground of my own home. My most sincere hope is that the knowledge contained in this book works as well for your children as it has for mine.

Bob Flaws
Boulder, CO

Table of Contents

1
An Introduction to TCM

I am a practitioner of Traditional Chinese Medicine (TCM). For the last 18 years I have specialized in the treatment of gynecological complaints. Because my patients are primarily women, once they see how effective Chinese medicine is for themselves, they often ask me to also treat their children. Thus I also have no little clinical experience caring for what in Chinese are called our little friends. In addition, I am always happy to treat children, not just because they are fun to be around, but also because Chinese medicine works so well for them. Further, as a parent myself, I know how important one's children's health is to a parent. Therefore, I have written this little book to share with other parents some of the wisdom of TCM when it comes to treating infants and children.

What is TCM?

TCM is that style of Chinese medicine taught at the approximately 30 provincial Chinese medical colleges in the People's Republic of China. Historically, this style stretches back over more than 2,000 years. Although TCM is in part based on Chinese folk medicine, TCM as a style is a highly sophisticated, literate, professional medicine. Its theories and practices have been developed and recorded by some of the most intelligent thinkers of Chinese society. It is estimated that there are approximately 30,000 volumes of existing Chinese medical literature written before the beginning of the twentieth century, while

1

thousands more have been published in this century alone. In addition, TCM journals in China publish approximately 100,000 articles per year, most of these being clinical audits on the effectiveness of certain treatments on certain diseases. So TCM is not just a folk medicine. Chinese medicine was a highly developed professional medicine when the West was still in the Dark Ages.

Does Chinese medicine work for Westerners?

China is a huge country, similar in many ways geographically to the United States. By this I mean that China stretches from the subarctic tundra in the north to the tropics in the south. It stretches from moist sea level in the east to the arid high altitudes of Tibet and Chinese Turkestan in the west. Its people are made up of more than 200 races, all of whom live, work, and eat differently. In other words, China itself is a very diverse place inhabited by a very diverse population, and Chinese medicine has been proven to work over the centuries throughout China.

In addition, TCM is the great rising star in the world of alternative and complementary medicines. Overseas-Chinese and non-Chinese practitioners now practice TCM in North, Central, and South America, in Europe, Africa, the Mideast, and Southwest Asia, and of course, Chinese medicine is practiced widely throughout all of Far East and Southeast Asia. In all these places, in all these climates, and in all these populations, Chinese medicine has been found to work. In fact, Chinese medicine works so well that the World Health Organization (WHO) has recommended TCM for worldwide propagation in the twenty-first century.

What's wrong with Western medicine?

It's true that Western medicine has done some very wonderful things in the last 150 years. However, Robert J. Samuelson, in a recent issue of *Newsweek* magazine (Jan. 8, 1996), quotes a study showing that, whereas 73% of Americans had a great deal of confidence in modern Western medicine in 1966, only 23% of Americans have that same confidence today. In the last 30 years, more and more people have become aware of the many side effects and short-comings of modern Western medicine. In particular, the overuse of antibiotics in children has led to some serious health problems, including the epidemic of pediatric ear infections and antibiotics' suspected role in the development of allergies. Any parent who has had a child receive repeated rounds of various antibiotics for ear infections with those infections returning over and over again should know that approach has its limitations. Like all human endeavors, Traditional Chinese Medicine also has its limitations. However, the wonderful thing is that TCM can often supply what's missing from modern Western medicine and vice versa.

What's so special about Chinese medicine?

Chinese medicine is the oldest, continuously practiced, literate, professional medicine in the world. It is used by one quarter of the world's population, and it is quickly establishing itself as the world's most respected professionally practiced alternative medicine. The reason why there is so much interest in TCM is not just that it works but also how it works. Modern Western medicine treats diseases. TCM works by restoring harmony and balance to the entire individual.

It is said in TCM,

Same disease, different treatments; Different diseases, same treatment.

What this means is that two patients may each suffer from the same named disease, for instance tonsillitis. However, in TCM, they may each be given radically different treatments. Conversely, two patients may each be suffering from different diseases, yet in TCM, they may both be given essentially the same treatment. This is because TCM practitioners treat patterns of disharmony and not just diseases. If two patients with the same disease exhibit different patterns of disharmony, they will receive different treatments. In other words, what works for the one might not work for the other or may even produce side effects because their overall pattern of disharmony is not the same. If two patients have different diseases but their patterns are identical, then they may be treated with the same treatment since their overall disharmony is basically the same.

We have all had the experience that some over-the-counter or even prescription medicine has worked for one of our friends or relatives but failed to work for us even though we had the same named disease or complaint. The reason the medicine did not work or even caused side effects is because our overall pattern of disharmony was not the same as our relative or friend's. When we are diagnosed with a disease, we must have a certain core group of signs and symptoms which are a defining part of that disease. For instance, someone with a headache has to have pain in the head. Otherwise we cannot say they have a headache. But even if two people both have pain in their heads, they may also have a number of other signs and symptoms which are not the same. It is these accompanying signs and symptoms, which Western medicine typically overlooks as a nonessential part of the diagnosis, that go to describe a person's Chinese pattern of disharmony.

It is a fundamental belief within TCM that all healing is based on the restoration of harmony and balance to the human organism. However, we are all out of balance in so many different ways. No one treatment can or will restore harmony and balance to everyone, even everyone with the same named Western disease. The greatest thing that TCM has to offer human beings throughout the world is a way of assessing each individual's own particular imbalance or disharmony, and, as an extension of that, a way of assessing exactly which medicines or treatments out of all others will bring that patient back to balance and health without either short or long-term side effects.

Why TCM especially for pediatrics?

Medicine is a very difficult art to practice. Even after two decades of study and practice, there are many things in the field of medicine I am not sure about. But when it comes to TCM pediatrics, I am absolutely sure that it holds the key to remedying the most common children's complaints and diseases. Although adult disease may be multifaceted and very difficult to diagnose and treat, most children's complaints revolve around a central key issue. Chinese medicine has the best discussion I know of this central or key issue at work in most children's complaints. Further, I have seen Chinese medicine achieve remarkable cures where rounds and rounds of antibiotics have failed. Thus I feel extremely positive in introducing Chinese medicine to parents as a way to help keep all our little friends healthy and well.

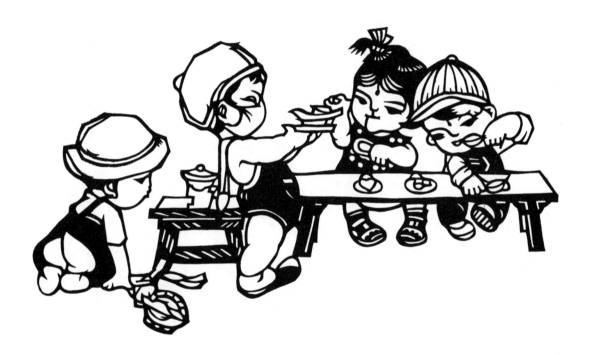

2
The Main Cause of Most Children's Diseases

In TCM pediatrics, it is believed that children are not simply miniature adults. Rather, children are immature physically and functionally according to Chinese medicine, and most of the common pediatric complaints are due to this immaturity. Describing children's physiology, it is said, "The viscera and bowels are tender and delicate and the form [*i.e.*, the body] and qi are not full." This saying which every TCM pediatrician learns by heart is supported by the following quotes from the Chinese medical literature. The *Ling Shu* or *Spiritual Pivot*, one of the two books of the *Nei Jing* or *Inner Classic*, the most famous Chinese medical classic, says, "Children's flesh is fragile, their blood scanty, and their qi weak." The *Zhu Bing Yuan Hou Lun (Treatise on the Origins & Symptoms of Various Diseases)* written around 650 AD states, "Children's viscera and bowel qi is soft and weak." Later, the *Xiao Er Yao Zheng Zhi (Essential Patterns & Treatments in Pediatrics)* says, "The five viscera and six bowels are made but not complete... are complete but not strong." And finally, the *Xiao Er Bing Yuan Fang Lun (Treatise on the Origins of Pediatric Diseases & Their Formulas)* says,

> "The skin and hair, muscles and flesh, sinews and bones, brain and marrow, the five viscera and six bowels, the constructive and defensive, and the qi and blood of children as a whole are not firm and secure."

Because of this inherent infirmity and weakness of children's bodies and organic function, it is also said, "Children are easily susceptible to disease which transmit and change rapidly." In particular, Chinese medicine holds that children are particularly susceptible to diseases associated with three main viscera, the lungs, the spleen, and the liver. The *Zhong Yi Er Ke Xue (The Study of Chinese Medicine Pediatrics)* says,

> "Children's exterior defensive function is not secure; therefore, external evils easily enter the exterior and assail the lungs."

This explains why children so often have upper respiratory tract complaints, such as colds, coughs, allergies, and asthma. The same book says,

> "Children's transportation and transformation function [*i.e.*, digestion or what is referred to as the spleen in Chinese medicine] is not fortified and complete; therefore they are easily damaged by food."

This explains why children so commonly suffer from colic, vomiting, diarrhea, indigestion, and stomachache. As we will also see below, there is a very close relationship in Chinese medicine between the spleen or digestion and the lungs, and even many upper respiratory tract complaints either begin in or are aggravated by faulty digestion in turn due to improper diet. Speaking of the liver, *Dan Xi Xin Fa (Dan-xi's Heart Methods)* says, in children "The liver commonly has a surplus." In Chinese medicine, the liver is associated with spasms and convulsions as well as emotional upsetment and, in particular, anger. This saying helps explain why children are so easily upset on the one hand and why, when they have high fevers, they may develop convulsions.

The good news is that Chinese medicine also says, "Their visceral qi is clear and effective; therefore they easily and quickly return to health." Because children's body's have not accumulated the years of metabolic wastes and because their viscera and bowels have not borne the brunt of years of insult and injury, when they get ill, children typically bounce back to health quickly and easily. This is a very important point to remember, and children's recuperation will be all the quicker if one understands the pivotal role of the spleen and diet in their illnesses and recovery.

Diet as the key cause of most children's diseases

In particular, children under the age of five or six are believed to have immature or weak digestion and it is this fact which accounts for most of the commonly encountered pediatric diseases, including colic, earache, cough, swollen glands, allergies, and pediatric asthma and eczema. In Chinese medicine, the digestion is spoken of as the spleen and stomach and it is a statement of fact that, "In children the spleen is insuffi-cient." This use of the words spleen and stomach is different from how Western biology uses these words, and I caution Western readers not to confuse these two uses. Unfortu-nately, I must translate these two terms from Chinese as spleen and stomach, but the reader should put aside most of what they may know of these organs based on Western biology.

The Chinese medical conception of digestion

According to TCM, the process of digestion is likened to the process of the distillation of alcohol. The stomach is likened to a fermentation vat. It receives the food and drink which are "rottened and ripened" in the stomach. However, this pot of the stomach sits on a stove. That stove is the spleen which provides the heat which drives off the essence of the food and drink the same way that fire under a still drives off the alcohol from the mash. This means that it is the warmth of the spleen which provides the force for the transformation of food and liquids. This warmth of the spleen is called the spleen yang when describing its warming function, while it is referred to as spleen qi when describ-ing its transforming and transporting function.

Thus the spleen yang qi transforms the finest essence of food and liquids into a vapor which it sends upward to the heart and lungs. This finest essence of food and liquids becomes qi in the lungs, while it becomes blood in the heart. The lungs then send the qi out to the rest of the body just as the heart sends the blood out to the rest of the body. The qi provides the motivational force for all other transformations and transportations in the body, while the blood provides the moistening and nourishment for all the tissues of the body. If the qi and blood are sufficient and flow freely and without impediment to the entire body, then there is the power to function and the nourishment to build and repair the body and also to fuel that function. If, however, there is insufficient qi and blood, then function and nourishment are weak and deficient and there is the possibility of disease.

The finest essence which becomes the qi and blood is like the essence of alcohol that is driven off to collect in the cooling coils of a still. In Chinese medicine, this finest essence is often simply referred to as the clear. In contradistinction, the dregs or what is left behind are called the turbid. Hence the creation of qi and blood out of the finest essence of food and drink is also described as the separation of clear and turbid. The clear is sent upward to become the qi and blood, while the turbid is sent downward to be excreted as waste from the body through urination and defecation.

As stated above, Chinese doctors believe that the baby's spleen and stomach or digestion is inherently weak and immature. This means that the baby's digestion has a hard time separating clear and turbid efficiently and completely. On the one hand, this means that, although the baby eats and drinks, they do not make the same amount of qi and blood an adult would. Thus the baby spends much more time sleeping than the adult. On the other hand, this means that turbid qi is not always excreted as efficiently as possible. Instead, this turbid material may collect internally and "gum up the works."

Phlegm, food & dampness

In Chinese medicine, this turbid material may collect in the stomach and intestines where it obstructs the free flow of the stomach and intestinal qi and depresses their function. This then causes abdominal distention, stomachache, constipation, diarrhea, and/or vomiting. This turbid material may also overflow from the middle burner or middle section of the body, the home of the spleen and stomach. Typically, this turbid residue is seen as damp in nature. Thus this turbid dampness may cause all sorts of symptoms associated with excess dampness, such as diarrhea and vomiting as well as damp skin lesions. If this dampness congeals, it may form phlegm.

According to Chinese medicine, phlegm is nothing other than congealed dampness resulting from incompletely digested food and drink. Because it is the spleen which is the motivating force for the separation of clear and turbid, *i.e.*, the digestion of food and drink, it is said, "The spleen is the source of phlegm production." However, phlegm, once it is produced, tends to accumulate in the lungs. This is supported by the saying, "The lungs are the place where phlegm is stored." If phlegm gathers in the lungs, it obstructs and inhibits the flow of lung qi and this results in stuffy nose, runny nose, sneezing, coughing, and even asthmatic wheezing.

The most commonly encountered pediatric diseases are either upper respiratory tract complaints, such as cough, cold, asthma, and allergies, or are digestive tract complaints, such as colic, diarrhea, stomachache, and vomiting. The first group of diseases all have to do with phlegm accumulating in the lungs, while the second group have to do with poor digestion. However, since according to Chinese medical theory, phlegm is a by-product of poor digestion, one can say that the root of all these complaints is, in children, due to their immature and, therefore, faulty digestions. This is why my first teacher of Chinese medicine, Dr. (Eric) Tao Xi-yu of Denver, was fond of saying that all pediatric diseases are due to indigestion.

Inflammation & upward counterflow

Although this sounds simplistic in English, it is supported by very sound medical theory in Chinese and this theory is actually rather complex. For instance, in Chinese medicine, qi is believed to be inherently warm. Qi is also what transports and transforms food and liquids. If qi fails to transport and transform these foods and liquids and a turbid residue gathers and accumulates, this may obstruct the free and normal flow of the qi. The qi builds or backs up. Since it is inherently warm, if the qi backs up abnormally, there will be an abnormal accumulation of heat in that part of the body and this pathological accumulation may manifest as inflammation. Thus dampness may become damp heat, stagnant food may become stagnant food and stomach heat, and phlegm may become phlegm heat.

If this qi builds up to a certain point, eventually it must go somewhere. If turbid dampness, food, and phlegm keep the qi from flowing normally and it builds up like gas in a balloon, eventually it must find some avenue of escape. Because qi is yang, it also has an inherent tendency to move upward. That means that if it builds up past a certain point, qi will tend to counterflow abnormally upwards. This may then produce hiccuping, burping and belching, vomiting, and/or coughing.

Therefore, one can see that the poor digestion associated with young infants and children under the age of five or six can not only produce excessive dampness and phlegm inside the body, but can also indirectly be associated with counterflowing qi and inflammatory heat. When one adds these two disease mechanisms to the list, one can see that weak digestion may play a part in even more of the diseases and symptoms associated with infants and children.

And further, it is the qi which protects the body from invasion by various pathogens in the external environment. In Chinese medicine, various pathological bacteria, viruses, and fungi existing outside the body are called external evils. If the spleen and stomach promote good, efficient digestion, sufficient qi and blood are manufactured and this sufficient qi defends the exterior of the body from these external evils or pathogens. If this qi is not manufactured in sufficient quantities, then the exterior of the body may be abnormally susceptible to invasion. Thus because babies have weak stomachs and spleens, they are also more easily invaded by external pathogens than adults. In layperson's terms, this means that they "catch" germs more easily.

The implications of the root of pediatric disease being weak or immature digestion

There are three main implications of the root of most common pediatric disease being weak or immature digestion. First and very obviously, if digestion plays such a pivotal role in the health and well-being of infants and young children, then diet is extremely important both in terms of preventing disease as well as in treating it. The following chapter is devoted to a discussion of diet and children's health. Secondly, treatment for most children's diseases should also pivot around regulating and strengthening digestion. As we will see below, when it comes to the TCM treatment of most of the commonly encountered children's diseases, attention to regulating and improving digestion is central. And third, because the spleen and stomach automatically mature around the age of six or so, most common pediatric diseases are self-limiting. This means that children automatically tend to out-grow them. This is an important point which laboring parents should keep in mind when they have lost sleep for the third night in a row due to a coughing son or a feverish, crying daughter with an earache.

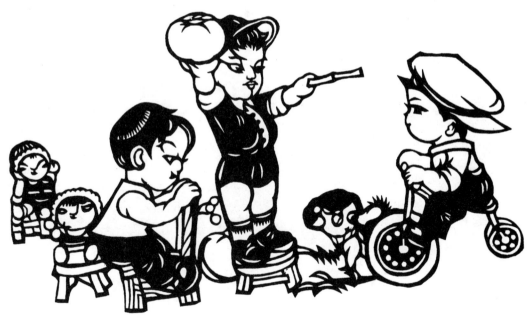

3
Chinese Dietary Therapy & Pediatrics

I believe so strongly in the truth of the above described Chinese theory regarding the spleen and stomach and children's diseases that I have gone to day-care centers to present free in-services trying to change the way we feed infants and toddlers. If our children suffer from a plethora of unnecessary runny noses, coughs, allergies, and earaches, which I believe they most certainly do, it is mainly because we, as a society in the West, have forgotten how to feed babies and young children. What the average Western parent has been led to believe is a healthy diet for infants and children is a dietary disaster according to TCM, and most pediatric diseases can be either completely eliminated or markedly relieved if one simply changes the child's diet.

Breast-feeding

Human breast milk is the single best food for babies. It is the right temperature and the right consistency. All other substitutes for human breast milk are second best. That being said, then why do even breast-fed babies develop colic, earaches, coughs, etc.? Typically, the first complaint of very young infants who are brought to my office is colic. Colic refers to stomach cramps with accumulation of gas which worsens in the afternoon and may continue on into the night. The baby cries until they can pass gas, and they typically demand to be carried, jiggled, or moved about. Colic is seen as a digestive complaint in TCM pediatrics. Essentially, it is due to food stagnation. This means that food is not transformed and transported properly by the spleen qi but rather gathers and obstructs the stomach and intestines.

Although human breast milk is the perfect food for human babies, even breast-fed children can develop colic. How can this happen? The answer is that too much of a good thing is still too much. In the last few decades, feeding on demand has become the norm. We have come to believe that feeding whenever the baby demands to be fed is somehow emotionally the right thing to do. However, when we feed on demand, we typically overfeed. When the stomach and spleen are inundated with more food than they can deal with efficiently and effectively, even human breast milk may become stagnant food and thus lead to digestive discomfort.

In Chinese, feeding on demand is called "unregulated feeding" and unregulated feeding is described as the disease cause of colic in the Chinese medical literature. The professional practitioner of TCM trained in pediatrics can tell if colic is due to overfeeding by the smell of the baby's breath, vomit, and stools and by the appearance of the vein at the base of the baby's index finger. When a child's colic or other disease is due to food stagnation, it is extremely important to stop feeding on demand and start feeding more or less on a schedule. If the child has just been borne, in order to protect the health of the child, it is important to initiate feeding on schedule, not on demand, right from the very beginning.

Feeding on schedule, not on demand

Scheduled feeding is what Western mothers used to do up until only two to three decades ago. Scheduled feeding, or what the Chinese call regulated feeding, does *not* mean starving the child nor does it mean being unkind. The baby is not any wiser than we adults. In fact, although the baby may be closer to its instinctual needs, it lacks the discipline and judgement of adults based on experience. The parent is in charge of the baby. The parent is supposed to know what is best for the baby better than the baby itself. Babies will feed out of boredom and out of gluttony just as adults do. If there is any single thing I would recommend to parents of newborn infants, it would be to breast-feed if at all possible but also to be sure to feed on schedule, not on demand.

If one goes to their local library, one will probably find a whole shelf of books on breast-feeding. Some of these books recommend giving the breast to every baby *every time the baby cries*. One of the rationales of breast-feeding on demand is that babies gain weight faster when fed on demand, but there is no discussion of the assumption that quicker weight gain is actually a good thing for the child long-term. Is it possible that the great rise in obesity among younger Americans is, at least partially, due to having been fed on demand so that they have become habituated to allaying every discomfort by eating something? Certainly proponents of the Japanese diet called Macrobiotics have long held that the increase in size and weight associated with post-World War II overeating and overnutrition is bad for one's health. As a simple guideline for scheduling feedings in newborns, one should consider a regimen of 2-3 ounces of milk every four hours. Although each individual baby has their own nutritional needs based on their own metabolism, this was the schedule that was recommended before breast-feeding on demand became the current dogma.

Feeding on schedule, not on demand, is considered anathema by many breast-feeding advocates. But I have been treating babies for almost two decades, both in the United States and in China, and I feel very positive that feeding on demand is one of the root causes of pediatric disease in the West. I believe that a return to scheduled feeding as opposed to feeding on demand could significantly decrease colic, earaches, and coughs and colds in infants. These conditions are, to a certain degree, causally related, and avoiding food stagnation and its subsequent colic can change a person's whole child-hood health history.

What to do if one cannot breast-feed?

Scanty lactation

If, after delivery, a woman finds that she has insufficient breast milk, she should drink some dark beer, such as a stout, should add papaya to her diet, and also regularly eat some ham, peanuts, and black sesame seeds. Chinese medicine believes that all these things can increase milk production. Malted barley can stop lactation when made into a tea, but malted barley brewed into beer seems to have the opposite effect, rather promoting lactation. Papaya strengthens the digestion and we have seen that the blood as well as the qi is manufactured by the spleen or the digestion. Ham, peanuts, and black sesame seeds are all believed to be very yin foods, and blood is categorized as a yin substance in Chinese medicine. Therefore, eating ham, peanuts, and black sesame seeds can increase blood and yin fluids. Chinese medicine also believes that pigs feet are a specific remedy for scanty lactation.

Recipes for scanty lactation

❶ Take 250g of day lily flowers (available at Oriental food stores) and 500g of pork. Soak the day lily flowers. Then stir-fry with the pork and some scallions and salt to taste. This nourishes the blood and frees the flow of the breast milk to treat scanty lactation.

❷ Take 2 pieces of tofu, 150g of towel gourd (available in Oriental food stores), 20g of mushrooms, and 1 pigs foot. Cut up the tofu, mushrooms, and towel gourd into pieces. Cook the pigs foot first by boiling it in water. Then add the tofu, mushrooms, and towel gourd and cook for 20 minutes longer. Add salt and fresh ginger to taste. This supplements the qi and blood and increases the secretion of breast milk.

❸ Take 60g of peanuts, 60g of yellow soybeans, and 2 pigs feet. First cook the soybeans and peanuts till soft. Add the pigs feet and cook into a soup. This supplements the spleen and nourishes the blood, opens the vessels and increases the milk.

❹ Cook a suitable amount of aduki beans into a porridge. This descends the qi and frees the flow of milk.

❺ Take 120g of brown sugar and 120g of fresh tofu. Boil together in water. Eat the tofu and drink the soup. This also supplements the blood and frees the breast milk. One can also add some rice wine (*i.e.*, mirin or sake) at the end to increase this recipe's efficacy.

❻ Cook 500g of papaya with 250g of fish and make into a soup. Add salt and fresh ginger to taste. One could also cook papaya with ham and peanuts.

❼ Make a tea by boiling 10g of anise in water. Add a little rice wine or sake and drink.

If the above simple remedies do not increase milk production, then the mother should try to find a professional practitioner of Chinese herbal medicine. There are many Chinese herbal formulas for increasing breast milk. However, because Chinese medicine works by restoring balance, it is important that the right formula be matched to the right pattern. Therefore, women wishing to use Chinese herbal medicine for the treatment of insufficient lactation should do so only based on a professionally supplied TCM pattern diagnosis. Over the years, I have successfully increased breast milk production in a number of women using Chinese herbal formulas.

Commercial formulas & other substitutes for human breast milk

However, if one cannot breast-feed for some other reason, what can one do? Obviously, one will have to use a "formula" or some other milk substitute. In Asia, the milk substitute that has traditionally been used is dilute rice soup. This is also the traditional first food other than the mother's breast milk introduced into the baby's diet. This food is nutritious and easy to digest. It is not so sweet as to create an addiction to the sweet flavor. It is also not so super nutritious that it creates excessive stagnant food, dampness, and phlegm. In addition, rice is warm in temperature and thus benefits the baby's digestion, or in Chinese parlance, their spleen and stomach yang.

Rice soup is made by putting rice and water in either a crock-pot or slow cooker at a ratio of 1 part rice to 6 parts water. This should then be cooked at a low heat for several hours or overnight. At the end of this time, what should be left is a very dilute rice soup, most of the rice starch having dissolved in the process of cooking. If this soup comes out too thick, one can simply add some more hot water to dilute it. Before pouring this soup into a baby bottle, one should strain out the remaining rice kernels through cheesecloth. To make rice soup for babies, one should use white rice which is more easily digestible than brown rice.

One can use cow or goat's milk as a human breast milk supplement for babies. However, since these milks are really not designed for the nutritional needs of human children, they can cause problems. In particular, if cow's milk is used, it should be watered down and not given whole. If using either commercial formulas, cow or goat's milk, or even the dilute rice soup described above, one should be careful not to give the child a bottle every time they cry. In other words, when feeding by a bottle, one should take even more care not to overfeed, thus causing food stagnation.

In particular, one should, in my experience, avoid either soy milk or soy-based formulas as substitutes for human breast milk. According to Chinese medical theory, soybeans are cold. Since the baby's spleen yang qi is itself weak, cold-natured soy milk can easily damage spleen yang and lead more quickly than other milk substitutes to food stagnation.

Further, one should not feed young babies fruit juices, such as apple juice or orange juice. These are too sweet and thus addicting. Anything that is sweet in flavor tends to engender dampness in the body and anything very sweet weakens the Chinese concept of the spleen. Western babies are typically given fruit juices because we think they are nutritious. In a sense they are. But they are super nutritious. They are more nutritious than what the baby actually needs. The intense sweet flavor creates a hankering or addiction on the one hand, while it engenders dampness and weakens the spleen on the other. Other than rice soup or dilute cow's milk, the only thing I recommend parents give their young babies is warm water if they think the baby is genuinely thirsty.

Introducing solid foods

Very young babies do not need anything other than breast milk and possibly a little additional warm water. However, somewhere around five to six months, the baby will start grabbing at food on the parents plates or on the dinner table. When the baby starts itself picking up food and putting it in their mouth, that is the time to begin introducing solid foods into their diet. This juncture is a very important cusp in the baby's development. How it is handled will determine much about the child's health for the next couple of years. The mistake that most Western parents make is introducing solid foods too early in the child's development, introducing too many different foods too rapidly, and introducing the wrong foods at the wrong times. If one introduces solid foods before the baby's digestion is ready to handle them, this will result in their non-transformation and thus the production of food stagnation, dampness, and phlegm. Therefore, it is extremely important to take one's cues from the baby itself.

100° soup

In order to understand even more clearly what Chinese medicine has to say about digestion and especially the child's digestion, one should keep in mind that everything the baby eats must be turned into 100° F soup before digestion can take place in the stomach. That means that food should be at the baby's body temperature or just a little above or below this. Most definitely the baby should not be fed chilled, iced, frozen, or cold foods. The process of digestion is a process of warm transformation based on the spleen's yang qi. Cold, chilled, and frozen foods weaken and even injure the digestion or spleen because they require so much yang qi to warm them up.

Secondly, food should be pureed so that it is like a thick soup. Babies do not have the back teeth which can mash food into a puree inside the mouth. Unless food is reduced to a mash, it cannot be digested in the stomach. Therefore, everything the baby is given should be cooked into a soup or blended in a blender or food mill.

Third, food should always be cooked. The process of digestion in Chinese medicine is a process of cooking food into soup. The more food is like a 100° soup when it is eaten, the easier it is to digest. Many people think that raw foods are more nutritious than cooked foods. However, this is only true in a sense. Uncooked foods do have more vitamins and enzymes than cooked foods. However, these nutrients are held within the walls of the cells. It is the cell walls that keep foods from being a formless puddle. These cell walls are like bags or boxes. In order to get at the nutrients, these bags and boxes must be broken down to get at the nutrients within. This is accomplished by chewing and by the digestive process. Because very young children do not have the teeth to chew efficiently and because their digestive processes are inherently weak and imma-ture, babies are not as efficient at breaking down these cellular bags and boxes as adults.

Cooking is another way humans break down the cellular bags and boxes that surround vital nutrients. Although cooking itself may destroy some of these nutrients, cooking makes the nutrients which are left much more easily assimilable. As an example, an uncooked carrot may have a hypothetical 100 units of some nutrient and a cooked carrot may only have 80 of those same units. If, however, one absorbs only 60 units from the uncooked carrot but 70 from the cooked carrot, the cooked carrot is still more nutritious than the raw carrot. This is the difference between gross nutrients and net absorption.

Cooking is nothing other than predigestion on the outside of the body. Cooking does some of the work of digestion before the food actually enters the stomach. Since babies' stomachs and spleens are weak and immature to begin with, they, even more than adults, benefit from the predigestion of cooking.

All this means that whatever the baby is given as their first food should be served warm, mashed or pureed, and cooked, not raw.

What to introduce when

The first food other than mother's milk should be the dilute rice soup described above. This engenders the qi, blood, and body fluids at the same time as it fortifies the spleen, harmonizes the stomach, and seeps out excessive dampness.

Because the baby is new to the world and everything in it, their tastes are not yet jaded. One does not have to vary babies' diets the same way an adult requires. This is good because it is very important that one introduce only a single new food at a time and that one continues feeding this food for some time before introducing another. By introducing one food at a time, one can see whether or not the child can actually digest that food. If the child's digestion is not yet mature and strong enough to digest that food without side effects, there will be some sign of indigestion, such as vomiting, colic, gas, constipation, or loose stools.

If one feeds a baby a new food and consequently there is some sign of indigestion, one should immediately suspend that food *for the time being*. One should wait a couple of weeks or even a month and then try the food again. If there are no signs of indigestion after one week, then it is safe to assume that the child's digestion is capable of handling that food and another food can be tested. If one misses such signs of indigestion as loose stools, constipation, and increased gas, then the undigested food will accumulate in the gut and transform into food stagnation, dampness, and phlegm. At that point, the manifestations will be increased mucus, either mucus in the stools or mucus in the nose and lungs. If one sees such increased mucus after having introduced a new food to the child's diet, once again they should suspend that food for a couple of weeks or even longer before trying it again.

If one introduces several foods at one time or does not allow a week between each new food introduced, one will not know what foods are causing what reactions. Therefore, it is important to go slowly and not rush this process. This is something like an elimination diet for those with allergies. In fact, by introducing foods in this way, one will avoid creating food allergies in their children. According to Chinese medicine, food allergies occur in children because they have been fed too much of difficult to digest foods. These then cause indigestion and the various disease mechanisms which spring from food stagnation, dampness, and phlegm as their root.

In general, after white rice, one should introduce various cooked vegetables. One can next try cooked, mashed carrots. After that, one can try mashed potatoes. Then one can try mashed green beans or peas. One should feed nutritious but easily digestible foods first. These should be nutritious, but not overnutritious. In general, cooked vegetables fill this requirement. Most cooked vegetables are somewhat sweet. They are not greasy, fatty, or too high in hard-to-digest proteins. Animal proteins, including cheeses, wheat products, and corn should be kept for later when the child's digestion has matured and become stronger. After all, cooked corn will even go through the digestive tract of many adults and remain in pieces.

In particular, wheat is considered cooling and dampening by nature in Chinese medicine. That means that it is more difficult to digest than rice and more likely to cause food stagnation. The Chinese medical classics are full of admonitions not to overeat sodden wheat products which may easily cause food stagnation and injure the spleen or the process of digestion.

What children should not eat

What babies and young children should not be fed are fruit juices, especially chilled juices out of the refrigerator. These are too sweet and they are too cold. They harm the digestion and cause accumulation of dampness and phlegm. Babies and young children should not eat too much bread. This also harms the spleen and gives rise to dampness and phlegm. Babies and young children should not eat raw vegetables or very much cheese, nor should they eat any but the smallest amounts of peanut butter. As mentioned above under scanty lactation, peanuts generate yin in the body. Dampness and phlegm are both yin. Peanuts are very hard to digest and phlegm-producing according to the logic of Chinese medicine. And children should not be given sweets and ice cream. Sweets damage the spleen and engender dampness, while ice cream is not only too sweet (the sugar), it is also too dampening (the eggs and cream), and too injurious to the spleen yang qi (the freezing cold).

In listing the common foods babies and children *should not be given*, many parents will immediately recognize the typical Western toddler's daily fare. Raw carrots and celery, pieces of cheese, crackers and bread, peanut butter and jelly, chilled milk and fruit juices. These are the foods we modern, rushed parents so often feed our children. They are also the staple diet at many day-care centers, where preparing and feeding cooked foods is too difficult. And this is also why our Western children get sick the way they do with earaches, allergies, and chronic coughs.

When parents bring a sick toddler to my clinic, whether with a common cold, tonsillitis, cough, or earache, my first question is whether or not they went to a birthday party right before they got ill. Four times out of five the answer will be yes. How did I know? Well, what do children eat at birthday parties? Sugar and ice cream. That is also why the weeks from Halloween through Christmas are the busiest time of the year for seeing pediatric patients.

How to keep your child from getting sick

As both a parent and a practitioner of Chinese medicine, my key advice for keeping your child healthy and well is to watch their diet and their poops. By watching their diet, I mean not feeding infants on demand, not introducing solid foods too early or too quickly, and not feeding raw, chilled foods. This also means not feeding too much dairy, meat, eggs, or greasy, fatty foods, and especially not feeding much in the way of sugars and sweets. What it does mean is a diet high in complex carbohydrates and high in vegetables with small amounts of meat, eggs, and dairy just like the Department of Agriculture's Food Pyramid. (See below.)

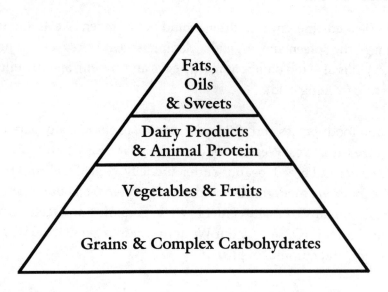

By watching your child's poop I mean that one can keep tabs on a child's diet by keeping an eye on their feces. If a young child's stools have become loose, it is often a sign that they have been eating too much sugar and sweets. It may also mean they have been eating too much ice cream, the single most delicious and dangerous food I know. When a child overeats sugars and sweets, including ice cream, this injures the spleen and causes the spleen to lose its control over the separation of clear and turbid. If the clear and turbid are not separated completely, dampness is engendered, and this dampness and undigested food flows downward in the form of loose stools or diarrhea. Typically, if one sees that a young child's stools have become loose due to faulty diet, one will then see a day or two later an increase in phlegm and mucus.

Once this increase in damp phlegm becomes apparent, then we say the child has caught a cold, has a runny nose or a wet cough, has swollen glands, or has an earache. In other words, based on my experience, first there is a lapse in dietary wisdom and control, then there are loose stools, and then the child gets sick. If one catches this progression when the stools have become loose but before increased phlegm and dampness have been generated, *and if one can get the diet back on track*, then one can reverse this disease process saving the child from becoming ill. Thus, by keeping an eye on babies' and toddlers' stools, one can adjust their diet before indigestion sets other disease processes in motion.

What to do about sugar & sweets

We all love sugar and sweets, and of course we all love to see the smile on children's faces when we give them something sweet to eat. It is such an easy way to make our little friends happy. And please be sure, I am not saying that we should never allow our little charges to eat a piece of candy, cake, or ice cream. This is not a perfect world and I am not counseling perfection in this regard. Of course we should allow our children to eat sweets from time to time. However, as their guardians, it is up to us to monitor the amount and to control this if it becomes excessive to the point of setting disease mechanisms in process.

As stated above, one can tell if the child's diet is within reasonable limits or not by their stools. If the stools are healthy and formed and the child is not producing a superabundance of mucus, then their diet is probably not too far out of line. If their stools get loose after eating sugar or ice cream, then it's time to tell the child that he or she cannot have that piece of candy or ice cream they are asking for. In other words, I am not talking about abstinence, but rather pacing. To never allow one's child to eat a piece of sweets would have its own harmful repercussions.

What if you've been feeding your child all wrong and they have developed some unfortunate addictions?

Many parents bring their children to acupuncturists and practitioners of Chinese medicine only after they have become ill. These children have become ill mostly because of faulty diet. By the time they make it into the office of a Chinese medical practitioner, they may already have become addicted to sweet foods and drinks. When the Chinese medical practitioner tries explain what a healthy diet is for the child, frequently the parent says that their child will not eat this or that. At that point, what's to be done?

There's the saying that, "Two wrongs don't make a right." If the child has become ill because of faulty diet, there is no way they are going to get well by continuing to eat the wrong foods. Just like with any addiction, there is going to be a period of "biting the bullet" and "going cold turkey." The child may refuse to eat the healthy food they are offered. They may cry and whine for what they are addicted to. But as long as the parents do not give in, eventually the child is going to eat. They may complain about it, they may make a fuss, but they will not starve themselves to death.

Unfortunately, such situations are not fun. But a mistake has been made and a correction is necessary. The child is by nature childish and cannot be expected to see the bigger picture and defer immediate gratification of their senses. But the parent is an adult and is the child's guardian. No matter how painful it is, it is the parent's duty to change the child's diet and see that they stick to this new, healthier way of eating. Everything passes and nothing lasts forever. Eventually the crying and stubbornness will give way to at least grudging compliance. On the other hand, the parent always has the option of letting the child eat what they want and continue to be sick. Each family has to make their own decisions. However, everyone needs to be clear that in such situations, one cannot have it both ways—a healthy child willfully eating sugars and sweets.

Conclusion

In the following chapter, we will discuss other ways to prevent disease and promote health according to the two thousand plus years of accumulated wisdom of Chinese medicine. However, I cannot overemphasize the importance of diet in young children's health. As my first mentor in Chinese medicine, Dr. (Eric) Tao Xi-yu, used to say, "Children only have one disease — indigestion." Of course, here we are not talking about congenital abnormalities, traumatic injuries, or unusual epidemic diseases. What

Dr. Tao was talking about was the common pediatric diseases of colic, cough, swollen glands, earaches, allergies, vomiting, diarrhea, and indigestion. Nine times out of ten, these are the things parents bring their children in to be treated for. Once these diseases have occurred, professional medical treatment may be needed remedially. But in the overwhelming majority of these cases, changes in diet can allow for natural and effective treatment and prevent their relapse.

The key points in Chinese dietary therapy for babies and young children are contained in the following verses. These are from *Pediatric Bronchitis: Its TCM Cause, Diagnosis, Treatment & Prevention* by Xiao Shu-qin *et al.* translated by Gao Yu-li and myself (Blue Poppy Press, 1991):

> Food and drink should be clear, light, and tasty;
> It should not be raw, cold, or greasy.
> It should be easy to absorb and assimilate, disperse and transform.
> Eat few tough, solid, difficult-to-digest foods.
> Be careful of sour, astringent, fishy smelling, and dry things.
> Do not eat more than the proper amount, stuffing oneself too full.

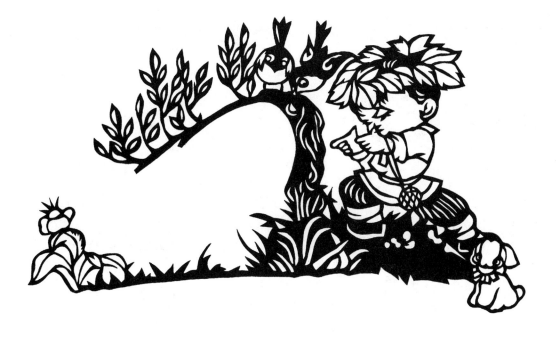

4
The Prevention of Disease & Promotion of Health

Chinese medicine since the time of the *Nei Jing (Inner Classic)*, the premier classic of Chinese medicine compiled approximately 2,500 years ago, has emphasized the prevention of disease before it arises. It is said in the *Nei Jing* that treating a disease once it has occurred is like digging a well after one has become thirsty or like forging spears after war has broken out. In English we would say it is like closing the barn door after the horse has run out. In Chinese medicine, there are several methods for preventing disease in children, the first and most important of which we have discussed above under diet and digestion.

Adequate rest & exercise

Because children's qi and blood are inherently weak and insufficient from the adults' point of view, they easily become fatigued. This is why children sleep so much. In Chinese medicine consciousness is due to the accumulation of yang qi. When this yang qi has been used up, we fall asleep in order to allow this yang qi to build back up again. Therefore, it is very important that children get enough rest. Often children will refuse to take a nap in the afternoon or refuse to go to bed on time. As harried parents, we may feel it is easier to give in to the child than to fight and argue and have to deal with their tears. However, if children get run down because of insufficient sleep, they become not only all the more unreasonable in their behavior but also more susceptible to disease.

On the other hand, it is also important that children get enough physical exercise. In Chinese medicine, exercise not only consumes qi and blood but also stimulates their production. This is because exercise benefits both the spleen and stomach and the heart and lungs. These are the viscera and bowels which are in control of the production of qi (stomach/spleen/lungs) and the production of blood (stomach/spleen/heart). Exercise improves the function of these viscera and bowels and thus benefits the production of qi and blood. If the qi and blood become full and exuberant, than evils or pathogens cannot enter the body easily and all the viscera and bowels receive the power and nourishment they need for healthy functioning. Therefore, it is important to regulate this yin/yang pair of adequate rest (inactivity/yin) with adequate exercise (activity/yang).

Fresh air

Fresh air is called the heavenly qi or great qi in Chinese. The qi within our body is made from the finest essence of food and drink distilled and transformed by our stomach and spleen combined with the great qi inhaled by our lungs. Germs can often build up in closed environments. Nowadays, in an attempt to conserve energy and be ecological, our homes are thickly insulated and our doors and windows are sealed. While this does cut down on energy consumption, it is still important that we get enough fresh air. Therefore, as long as the external environment is not too polluted, children should be encouraged to play outside where they can fill their lungs with fresh air.

Not too many clothes

Perhaps this next admonition is more germane for Asian parents who tend to swaddle their children thickly in clothes so that they often look like they can hardly move. In Chinese medicine, it is believed that children's constitutionally are very yang. What this means is that they typically require less clothes than adults for the same weather. If they wear too many clothes, their defensive mechanisms will not develop properly and they will tend to be too susceptible to invasion by external pathogens. They become like hot-house plants that do not have good resistance. To continue this gardening metaphor, when one grows seedlings in the spring, usually one leaves them out during the days and brings them in at nights before actually planting them in the ground. This is called hardening off. Children, likewise need to be hardened off. This does not mean, however, that children should not wear warm clothes when necessary. It only means that they should not be over-bundled.

Massage

Massage in China seems to have undergone a period of great flourishing and development in the Ming dynasty (1368-1644). During this time, many therapeutic massage manuals were published in China. Among these were a number on pediatric massage. In Chinese, pediatric massage is called *xiao er tui na*. Pediatric massage forms a part of the training of all doctors specializing in massage therapy in China and most TCM practitioners specializing in pediatrics will know the rudiments of this system. As we will see in the following chapter, there is a whole system of the remedial treatment of pediatric disease using this *xiao er tui na*. However, there are a couple of techniques every parent should learn.

Spinal pinch pull

This technique is used as preventive medicine in many Chinese day-care centers. It is believed to tonify all the body's viscera and bowels as well as to stimulate and regulate the central nervous system and the body's defensive exterior. It is usually done one time per day, every day, on infants and toddlers. One begins with the child laying naked on its stomach. One lightly grasps the skin lying over the child's sacrum between their thumbs and fore and middle fingers, gently but firmly pinching up this relatively loose skin. One then rolls this fold of skin upward slowly but steadily from the sacrum to the base of the neck. This rolling is accomplished by lifting the skin and then pushing the thumbs forward at the same time as pulling the fore and middle fingers back.

When one reaches the base of the neck, the hands leave the skin and return again to the sacrum to pinch up a new fold of skin. One does *not* reverse this maneuver and do it downward. *It is only done from sacrum upward to the base of the neck in one direction only.* The skin is rolled upward right over the center of the child's spine. This maneuver is repeated 3-5 times each session, not more. If this is done every day routinely, it is believed to improve the child's general state of health and their resistance to disease.

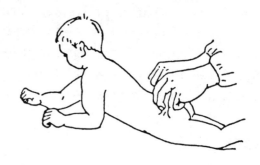

Rubbing the abdomen

We have already seen how important the digestion is to a baby or toddler's health and well-being. Therefore, it should come as no surprise that massaging the abdomen is an important way to help regulate and benefit the digestion. One begins with the child laying on their back with their abdomen exposed. One can rub with the flat fingertips of their dominant hand. Begin on the lower right abdomen and make small circles with the fingertips while sliding the hand slowly upward. The fingertips should remain in contact with the skin at all times. The pressure should be firm, yet gentle. This should not be uncomfortable for the child.

When the hand comes to the top of the abdomen, still making small circles, one continues across the top of the abdomen from right to left. When one reaches the left side of the upper abdomen, one changes direction and makes small circles downward. Upon reaching the lower abdomen on the lower left side, one can circle over to the right and continue up again on the right side. Thus one circles the entire abdomen from the right side up and over to the left, then down and over to the right again. This large circle follows the direction of the large intestine. Because the hands are moving around the abdomen by making smaller circles, I like to refer to this maneuver as making small circles within large circles.

Now the question should immediately arise, "What direction should the small circles go?" They can either circle to the right or the left, although most right-handed people will instinctively circle to the right if not told otherwise. The question what direction should the small circles go is an important one, since depending on the direction, this maneuver can have opposite effects. If one makes small circles to the right, this promotes defecation and the elimination of stagnation. Thus small circles to the right are good for excess conditions, food stagnation, and constipation due to accumulation. These small circles to the right help to drain the stomach and large intestine. If one makes small circles to the left, this strengthens the spleen and stops diarrhea due to spleen qi weakness and insufficiency.

So then the next question is, "How do I know if my child has a stomach and intestinal excess or a spleen deficiency?" and that is an excellent and intelligent question. In general, if your child has cold hands and feet, if they tend to be listless and fatigued, if they have a poor appetite and loose stools, and if they have an easily visible blue vein at the bridge of their nose and between their two eyes, they probably are spleen deficient and can benefit from these small circles to the left.

If, on the other hand, your child typically has a red face, has warm hands and feet, tends to be more constipated than loose, cries loudly and is very active, and if they have bad breath and foul-smelling stools, then they probably have a tendency towards stomach excess and food stagnation. These children benefit more from making the small circles to the right.

As we discussed in chapter one, in Chinese medicine, health is balance. Too much of even a good thing is bad. Therefore, readers should not think that tonifying the spleen is necessarily good if their child actually is suffering from a stomach excess and food stagnation. In that case, the best thing that you can do to restore health is not to make

35

the spleen stronger but to drain the excess
accumulation. So please do not think that
making circles to the left is inherently better
than making circles to the right. It is my
experience that in the West, more children
need the small circles to the right than to the left.

This rubbing of the abdomen should be done
several times a session. It is good to do this at least
one time per day in infants beginning even only a
day or two after birth and continuing up to around
one year. As we will see in the following chapter, this
is a very important technique for treating colic, and it can
be done anytime in the day if the child is suffering some digestive distress.

In general, massage is great for babies. It improves their digestion and elimination, it
stimulates the flow of blood and lymph, it exercises and stretches their muscles, and it is
a great way to bond with one's child. One can massage their entire baby every day. Dr.
Fan Ya-li, a Chinese doctor specializing in Chinese massage, gives a preventive full-body
infant massage routine in her *Chinese Infant Massage Therapy* also published by Blue
Poppy Press.

Treating early

Children should be treated, either at home or professionally, at the very first sign of
disease. That means that if the infant or toddler's stools become loose, the diet should
immediately be "tightened up." Usually, loosening of the stools is one of the very first
indications that the child is going to get ill due to eating the wrong foods. These are
most commonly sugars and sweets, including fruit juices, fatty, greasy foods, and raw,
chilled, cold, and frozen foods. If the stools get loose because the child has been allowed

to overindulge in these kinds of foods, then the first line of defense is to make sure these foods are taken out of the child's diet.

If one misses the loosening of the stools as typically the first sign that the child's health may be slipping, then the second sign is often an increase in nasal mucus. As soon as nasal mucus is seen, then again the parent should attend to their child's diet, making sure that the child is eating a clear, bland diet of cooked, warm foods and that they are not eating any sugar, sweets, raw, chilled, or frozen foods, or dairy products. At this point, the parent may rub the abdomen with the direction of the small circles depending on whether the child has cold hands and feet, a pale face, and a blue vein at the root of the nose between the two eyes, or has warm hands and feet, a red face, and a tendency to high fevers. In the former case, then the small circles should go counter-clockwise in order to help strengthen the spleen, while in the latter case, these small circles should go clockwise in order to help lead away stagnant food. In addition, professional practitioners will often prescribe various Chinese herbal formulas whose ingredients are meant to eliminate food stagnation, dry dampness, and transform phlegm. If the child tends to run cold, then spleen-strengthening ingredients are typically included, but if the child tends to run hot, then heat-clearing herbs may be added.

Chinese herbal medicine

Chinese herbal medicine is one of the most sophisticated herbal medicines in the world. Typically, combinations of six to 20 ingredients are used in formulas correlated to each individual's pattern of disharmony. Chinese herbal medicine is great for both preventive and remedial treatment with kids. Some people think Chinese herbal medicine is difficult for babies and toddlers to swallow. That would be true if they needed to swallow large amounts of bitter decoctions. However, children generally respond to very small doses. Therefore, one can give Chinese herbal medicine which has been decocted or boiled into a "tea" by using an eye-dropper and children will take this without spitting it out. Whereas the same child might very well refuse to drink the same tea when presented in a cup.

There are a number of formulas that have been used by Chinese doctors for literally two thousand years for improving the general health of children. Typically, these formulas consist of Chinese herbs which fortify the spleen, harmonize the stomach, eliminate dampness, transform phlegm, and clear abnormal heat from the stomach and intestines. One such formula is called in Chinese *Xiao Chai Hu Tang* (Minor Bupleurum Decoction). This is the most common formula I prescribe for preventive therapy for toddlers and young children. It can prevent chronic tonsillitis, chronic earaches, and chronic coughs and colds. However, it must be prescribed by a properly trained professional practitioner of Chinese herbal medicine. Parents should not prescribe this on their own. In fact, there are a number of other formulas which might be the correct one instead to bring your particular son or daughter back to balance.

I do not recommend every child take a Chinese herbal tea preventively. For most children, paying attention to diet is usually sufficient. However, when children have a history of chronic and recurrent infections which have been repeatedly treated by antibiotics, then using a Chinese herbal tea makes great sense. Typically, I begin these in the early fall and continue their administration through spring. In most cases, a single year of such therapy is enough to get the child back on track again. In only a few cases will such treatment need to be repeated an entire second year. This mostly occurs when the diet has not been sufficiently corrected or when more antibiotics have been used.

Is Chinese herbal medicine safe?

Recently there has been concern voiced in the popular media about the safety of Chinese herbal medicine. There have been reported cases of side effects and contamination of Chinese herbal products with heavy metals and even Western drugs. In general, I do not recommend parents purchase so-called Chinese patent medicines over the counter at either Chinese apothecaries in Chinatowns or at health food stores. It is true that some of these ready-made or patent medicines are contaminated by heavy metals, such as lead, while others contain aspirin, caffeine, and even prescription drugs which are not disclosed on their labels. Many Chinese patent medicines are high quality products with safe and effective ingredients and without adulteration or contamination. But how is a person to know which ones are safe and which ones should be avoided. Therefore, the simplest way to be sure is to avoid using such ready-made patent medicines manufactured in Asia where companies do not have to meet the more stringent manufacturing and labeling requirements we have in the West. (A few exceptions to this recommendation are given in the chapter on the treatment of various diseases.)

The Chinese herbal medicine that I am recommending is the use of bulk dispensed herbal medicinals which are then made into a "tea" or decoction. When such medicinals are dispensed in bulk, the practitioner has control over the quality and authenticity of each ingredient. Further, the practitioner can write an individualized prescription to fit your child's immediate and personal needs. When Chinese herbal medicines are prescribed in bulk form by trained professionals according to a TCM pattern discrimination or diagnosis, then Chinese herbal medicine is extremely safe and without side effects.

Some Western practitioners of Chinese medicine also use Western manufactured ready-made medicines, either in pill, powder, or tincture form. These are made from herbs grown or gathered in China or Taiwan but then are processed and manufactured in the West according to GMP or good manufacturing procedures. These pills, powders, and tinctures manufactured in the West using Chinese herbs are high quality, safe, and effective products whose ingredients are routinely screened by various laboratory tests to insure their purity, ingredients, and active constituents. Typically, these products are not sold over the counter in health food stores but only by prescription from trained professional practitioners.

Acupuncture

Acupuncture means the insertion of fine, sterile, stainless steel needles into certain points on the body in order to rebalance and bring harmony to the flow of qi and blood in the body. In general, acupuncture is not a main modality in pediatrics within Chinese medicine. Either it is used sparingly for remedial treatment or is avoided altogether by some schools of thought until after seven or even 13 years of age. However, acupuncture in a broader sense does include within its bag of tricks a number of related treatments which do not require the actual insertion of needles and which are very useful for treating children both preventively and remedially.

In Japan, a style of pediatric acupuncture was developed which is called *shonishin*. This is the Japanese pronunciation of the Chinese *xiao er zhen*, pediatric needle. However, the tools of *shonishin* hardly look like the typical acupuncture needle. Rather they are a collection of scrapers, combs, rollers, blunt probes, and brushes. Practitioners use these instruments to stimulate various acupuncture points and channels on the surface of the child's body. Thus these practitioners are able to stimulate and balance the child's qi without piercing the skin. In Chinese pediatrics, there is the saying, "Because of delicate and tender flesh and muscles, they transmit changes easily." On the one hand, this means that children transmit disease changes and pathogens easily through their body once infected. On the other hand, this also means that healing effects can also be more easily transmitted through the surface of the child than through the adult. Hence one can get the same or similar degree of stimulation with infants without necessarily piercing the skin.

Regular, weekly *shonishin* treatments can be a very effective means of both treating and preventing the recurrence of disease in children who suffer from chronic coughs, tonsillitis, and earaches. Once the condition is brought under control, parents may only chose to have their children *shonishin*ed every several months, similar to having the oil changed in one's car every 3,000 miles. Children typically love this treatment since it is very soothing and comfortable. However, not all acupuncturists are trained in this art, so ask beforehand.

Love & discipline

Most Chinese books on pediatrics do not say anything on these topics. Perhaps they are taken for granted. Here in the busy West where everyone tends to work outside the home, love and discipline cannot always be taken for granted. No child can flourish and be truly healthy in body and mind without a huge amount of love. This love needs to be expressed physically and verbally. Children also need clear-cut and consistent boundaries in order to feel secure. Love and discipline may seem like contradictory concepts, but children do not grow healthy and strong without the both of these working hand in hand.

Trying to keep your child healthy the natural way is not always the easiest way. A number of years ago there was an advertisement that said, "You can't fool Mother Nature." Sometimes after a busy day, allowing the child to eat whatever it wants may be the path of least resistance. But if the child gets an earache, staying up all night is surely no fun. Then going to the Western MD and getting antibiotics may seem like the path of least resistance. But recurrent earaches and trips to the ER are surely an even greater pain. If, through ignorance and the best of intentions, one has started out wrong and childhood health problems, such as recurrent tonsillitis or recurrent earaches, have become established, it may seem very difficult to break bad habits and to establish new, healthy ones. However, I can assure you, once one gets over the hump at the beginning, everything will get easier and easier.

Avoidance of antibiotics if possible

Antibiotics are wonderful, life-saving medicines when used correctly and in moderation. Unfortunately, antibiotics have been irresponsibly over-prescribed and erroneously prescribed for conditions which they cannot treat, such as viral infections. This has led to the development of many new strains of infectious bacteria which are resistant to antibiotic treatment. However, even if that were not the case, antibiotics should be reserved for the few cases in which they are truly necessary. This is because antibiotics

41

are so powerful. Not only do they kill disease-producing bacteria, but they commonly kill off the good bacteria upon which our health is founded.

Our bodies are home to many bacteria which actually work for us in healthy ways. In particular, our digestive tracts are homes to all sorts of bacteria and fungi which are commensal, meaning they live within our house, and which are symbiotic, meaning that both sides benefit from their presence. These bacteria help break down foods and the waste products of digestion. Others of these bacteria help keep populations of various yeast and fungi in proper proportions. These yeast and fungi also live within us symbiotically and provide us with certain necessary services.

If, however, antibiotics wipe out these healthy bacteria along with disease-producing ones, it upsets the balance of power within our system and especially within our guts. This then sets in motion a series of events which have profound negative repercussions on our long-term health and well-being. If the bacteria which keep the yeasts and fungi in our intestinal tracts under control are harmed, these populations explode. When they do, they do three important things. First, they invade the interior of the body by moving out of the intestinal tract (which is technically still the outside the body). Once inside the body, they must protect themselves from attack by the body's immune system. After all, these now are foreign cells which should not be inside the body. In order to defend against the host body's immune response, these yeasts and fungi very cleverly manufacture and release certain hormone-like substances that: 1) weaken the immune system, making it less efficient, and 2) upset the delicate balance between the various hormones of the body. These hormones are the messengers of the body which help keep the body's homeostasis healthy and normal.

Secondly, eventually these yeasts and fungi die. When they die, they break down into foreign molecules. The body's immune system recognizes these foreign molecules as foreign and mounts an immune response or attack. Thus, although these yeasts and fungi weaken the immune system by confusing it, they also cause it to be perpetually fighting their breakdown products.

Third, when these yeasts and fungi move through the intestinal wall, they allow the intestinal wall to become permeable to other things which should not be allowed into the interior of the body. This is called "leaky gut syndrome." These other things are large, undigested molecules of food. If these get into the interior of the body, the body's defense or immune system recognizes these large, undigested food molecules as foreign and so also mounts an immune response or attack. Thus the body becomes allergic to these large food molecules passing undigested through the gut, since an allergy is nothing other than an immune response to a substance which, in healthy people, does not normally cause an immune reaction.

Therefore, the net result of killing off the healthy bacteria in our guts by wrong or repeated use of antibiotics will lead to: 1) leaky guts, 2) hormonal dysregulation of the immune system, and 3) perpetual allergic responses. These perpetual allergic responses eventually exhaust the immune system, making the host more and more susceptible to germs it would ordinarily take care of without symptoms of disease. Finally, the body's immune system get so overworked and so out of balance that it loses all sense of what is foreign and what is self. At that point it may even start attacking itself and cause auto-immune diseases, such as rheumatoid arthritis, multiple sclerosis, and lupus erythema-tosus.

This scenario is involved in the disease mechanisms of most of the diseases with which people in developed countries are more and more concerned: allergies, immune deficiencies, and autoimmune diseases, but also many viral conditions, including diabetes. As a TCM gynecologist, I also see this scenario playing a part in endometriosis, immunological infertility, and even PMS and menopausal syndrome through autoim-mune thyroiditis and ovaritis. This scenario even plays its part in development and progression of many cancers. Therefore, this scenario is a key one in understanding and successfully treating a whole host of diseases, including chronic, recurrent earaches, chronic, recurrent tonsillitis, and chronic allergies, including eczema and allergic asthma, in children.

Chinese medicine & antibiotics

For the last several paragraphs, I have been talking about antibiotics and their side effects in terms of Western biology. However, Chinese medicine has its own description of these same events. In Chinese medicine, herbs which have pronounced antibacterial, antimicrobial, anti-inflammatory abilities are usually described as being very "cold." This is because most microbial infections result in some sort of inflammation. Such symptoms of inflammation are seen as the pathogenic or evil presence of heat in the body. Since cold is what clears heat, medicinals which have pronounced antimicrobial, anti-inflammatory effect on the body are described as being cold in nature.

The logic of this description is supported by another factor. Since digestion in Chinese medicine is believed to be a process of warm transformation, excessively cold medicinals may damage this process. In Chinese medicine this is described as damaging the spleen. If the spleen becomes damaged by wrong or overuse of cold, anti-inflammatory medicinals, then the symptoms that appear are various digestive complaints such as diarrhea and loose stools and gas and abdominal distention after eating. These are exactly the kinds of side effects many antibiotics have. Because the spleen in Chinese medicine is associated with the production of healthy or righteous qi in the body, damage to the spleen also results in fatigue, cold hands and feet, reduced appetite, and a pale or sallow complexion. Further, because the righteous qi is what fights evil or pathogenic qi in the body, if the spleen becomes weak, the body cannot fight off invasion or infection as efficiently as it should. Thus it is said in Chinese medicine that assailing evils take advantage of this deficiency and repeatedly enter the body. In addition, because the spleen is responsible for the transportation and transformation of body fluids and liquids in the body, if cold medicinals damage spleen yang qi, water and dampness accumulate and transform and congeal into phlegm.

Therefore, one can see that even from the Traditional Chinese Medicine point of view, wrong or overuse of antibiotics can lead to damage of the spleen with repeated susceptibility to disease, such as earaches, tonsillitis, and various allergies, and the abnormal production and accumulation of phlegm and mucus, *i.e.*, colds, coughs, and asthma. If the spleen is strong, a person may be treated with antibiotics and bounce back quickly without much in the way of side effects or lingering repercussions. But if the spleen is weak or if antibiotics are used repeatedly, the spleen is weakened even further. Thus infections recur, more antibiotics are given, and the circle goes round and round and round.

The implications of this are that antibiotics should only be used when they are truly necessary. Just two days ago (January 16, 1996), a spokesperson for the American Medical Association went on TV and asked physicians the same thing — not to prescribe antibiotics unless truly necessary. The AMA may have a different interpretation of what is truly necessary, but at least some Western MDs are waking up to the fact that wrong and overuse of antibiotics is creating a major health care problem in the world.

I believe that antibiotics should be seen as the top rung on a ladder of graduated responses. If there is an infection, one should first try to use weaker, less drastic methods of treatment. If those do not work, one should then work their way up this ladder of graduated responses. If the condition is truly serious and potentially life-threatening or if there is the *likelihood* (not just the outside chance of serious, long-term damage), then yes, that is the time that antibiotics are truly and correctly warranted. In other words, antibiotics should be held as the trump card in case other treatments with less side effects fail. They are there, held in reserve to be used if necessary, but used *only* when necessary.

My own son's case

I would like to share with readers the story of my own son. When he was a baby, he was breast-fed and massaged every day. He had a touch of colic, but that did not last long nor was it very serious. It responded well to abdominal massage and some Chinese herbal medicine. We did not have him immunized at three months, but at six months, because we planned on traveling in Asia, we thought he should receive the usual vaccinations. He got one shot and immediately fell ill with an earache. Since he had never been ill until then, we immediately decided not to get him immunized further *and not to go to Asia at that time.* We treated his earache and fever with Chinese herbal medicine, massage, eardrops, and warm compresses, and he bounced back quickly. Over the next 10 years, he was never immunized and never took any antibiotics. We watched his diet and poops as described in the preceding chapter. When he got ill, which was not frequently, we treated him by adjusting his diet, sometimes using acupuncture, and often using Chinese herbal medicine — even the time he developed a mild case of scarlatina. When he was 10 or 11, he developed an acute staphylococcus infection in the bones of his hip and he required emergency surgery and a few weeks of very strong antibiotics. In his case, this infection seems to have been due to fetal toxins since he had no cuts or scratches which were infected nor was he sick in any other way at the time of this occurence. In any case, he bounced back from this much quicker than any of his doctors anticipated. He is now in eighth grade and, except for that episode and a recent one day cold, he has never missed a day of school for illness and he does not have any allergies.

I attribute my son's exceptional health history to date to: 1) his overall healthy diet and 2) to his lack of antibiotic experience. His lack of immunizations may also have contributed to his extremely good health, but that is very hard to say for sure. Nevertheless, when he really needed antibiotics, of course we used them. Otherwise he would have suffered permanent damage to his hip joint and may have even died. Chinese medicine cannot treat acute septicemia the way antibiotics can. Therefore, I strongly recommend that parents avoid antibiotic use as much as possible. In the following chapter, we describe many treatments which can be used as the lower rungs on the ladder of graduated responses I have described above. In actual clinical practice, antibiotics should be used as the exception rather than as the rule, and, combined with the dietary guidelines described above, avoidance or only a very sparing use of antibiotics is one of my key and crucial recommendations to parents.

Avoidance of immunizations, perhaps

Many parents assume that having their children immunized is unquestionably the correct thing to do. However, there is a growing body of literature that proves there are real risks with routine vaccinations. Some of these risks, such as death due to anaphylactic shock, are immediate and catastrophic. Other of these risks consists of possible lifelong damage and disease. Further, statistics do not confirm that the death rate for some of the diseases for which we regularly immunize went down *because of* immunization. In some cases, these rates seem to have declined even before immunization was adopted or simultaneously declined in societies that did not adopt immunization. Further, there are very real questions about how effective these vaccines are in providing immunity against these diseases. The U.S. Congress has created a Vaccine Injury Compensation Program for the compensation of victims suffering from side effects of immunizations. So it is absolutely clear and uncontestable that there is a risk to be run in getting vaccinated. Otherwise there would be no reason to have a compensation program. In other words, the whole subject of immunizations is a tricky one, and there are many parents who are confused about whether or not to immunize.

Since it is not clear to me that immunizations do not have long-term health consequences and since we know that a certain percentage of children *will* be seriously harmed by prophylactic immunizations, I generally counsel against them. However, this must remain the parents' decision and it is a decision with no perfect answers. In other words, one runs certain risks whether one does or does not immunize. Since this is not a perfect world and "nobody gets out alive", this should not be a surprising situation. But parents want only the best for their children and want to protect them against every possible harm. Unfortunately, we cannot do that, and often, trying to do that creates its own problems.

DPT

DPT stands for diphtheria, pertussis, and tetanus. Hence the DPT shot is a combination immunization against these three diseases. This is one of the very first immunizations a baby usually gets, receiving the first shot as young as two weeks of age. Although these three immunizations are usually given as a single injection, depending on one's locale and the willingness of the physician, one can get one or more of these shots by themselves. For instance, one can get just a tetanus shot or one can get a DT shot.

Diphtheria

Diphtheria is a very virulent and dangerous disease. However, in developed countries in the West, it is very rare. If one lives or travels in countries where diphtheria is a present danger, then immunization makes sense. Otherwise, I do not believe it is necessary. If an outbreak or epidemic was moving towards one's place of residence, then one should get this vaccine. Unfortunately, an FDA-sponsored vaccine review has concluded that "for several reasons, diphtheria toxoid, fluid or absorbed, is not as effective an immunizing agent as might be anticipated." Chinese medicine does treat this disease. However, it should be treated with a combination of Chinese and Western medicine, not just Chinese medicine alone.

Pertussis

Pertussis is also called whooping cough. It does exist within developed Western societies. However, pertussis is rarely lethal, while the pertussis vaccine sometimes is. The Institute of Medicine (IOM) of the National Academy of Science, comprised of 11 leading pediatricians in the United States, has spent 20 months reviewing hundreds of scientific studies on the safety and efficacy of immunizations. This panel concluded that the pertussis vaccine can cause a number of health problems. In addition, the Vaccine Advisory Committee of the U.S. Congress has produced a wealth of data about recurring problems with this vaccine. This vaccine was created in 1912 and has not been changed since. This vaccine has never been tested for safety in the U.S. and especially has never been tested for safety at the current dosage in children as young as six weeks of age or younger. The statistics also do not prove that this vaccine works particularly well in preventing this disease. In recent outbreaks of whooping cough, half or more of all sufferers had been fully vaccinated. According to Prof. Gordon Stewart writing on the pertussis vaccine in *The Lancet*, "No protection by vaccination is demonstrable in infants." While Dr. Morris, testifying before the Subcommittee on Investigations & General Oversight in May 1982 stated that pertussis vaccination has only been shown to be *between* 63-93% effective.

Chinese medicine does treat pertussis. Therefore, I do not advise taking the risk of the pertussis vaccine when effective Chinese medical treatment is possible. If, however, professional Chinese medical treatment is not locally available, one should also take that into account when making a decision about this vaccine.

Tetanus

Tetanus infection is usually the result of an unclean puncture wound or cut. It is caused by germs which live in dirt. Unless a wound is contaminated by contact with dirt, tetanus is not very likely. According to Dr. Velia Hempel of Germany, the immunity provided by tetanus shots wears off after 10 years. In the U.S., if one gets a serious cut requiring medical attention, the doctor will want to give a "booster" shot in any case. According to Dr. Hempel, such booster shots are not given in Europe and cannot provide any immunity for a cut which has already occured since it takes a number of days before immunity is established. That means that all adults who think they have a lifetime immunity to tetanus are wrong. Again according to Dr. Hempel, this is the same situation with most other immunizations — they do not confer lifetime immunity; their effect wears off. This raises a very large question, at least in my mind. It means that most of us probably do not have the immunity that we think we do. Although Chinese medicine does have treatments for tetanus, it should be treated by a combination of Chinese and Western medicines.

The Institute of Medicine (IOM) study cited above has concluded that the DPT vaccine *definitely* can cause numerous health problems, including death. There is evidence that "indicates a causal relation" between administration of this vaccine and anaphylactic shock. Anaphylactic shock is an extreme allergic reaction which, if not treated immediately can lead to death. This same study found that this vaccine also caused extended periods of inconsolable crying and screaming lasting up to 24 hours. Harris L. Coulter and Barbara Loe Fisher in *DPT: A Shot in the Dark* say this crying resembles the so-called *cri encephalique* which accompanies some cases of encephalitis. Encephalitis or meningitis, an inflammation of the brain, may result in either permanent brain damage or death, and the IOM study did find a link between DPT vaccinations, acute encephalopathy, and shock. A group called Dissatisfied Parents Together (DPT) believes their children have been permanently harmed in this way by this vaccine. Other possible side effects of the DPT vaccine are chronic neurologic disease, Guillain-Barre syndrome (a type of paralysis), juvenile diabetes, learning disabilities, attention deficit disorder (ADD), infantile convulsions, and sudden infant death syndrome (SIDS). From January through August of 1991, the Vaccine Adverse Event Reporting System set up by the Compensation Act received 3,447 reports of DPT reactions. Included were 398 cases of convulsions, 218 cases of shock, 72 cases of febrile seizures, and 75 cases of sudden infant death syndrome. Thus clearly there are risks associated with the DPT shots which every parent must carefully weigh before having their child immunized.

Polio

Mine was the first generation mass immunized against polio. Growing up I had a friend who had one leg smaller than the other because of atrophy due to polio. I have also seen many polio patients in Chinese hospitals. So I know polio is real. If one lives in a developed Western country, the incidence of polio is rare. However, the vaccine itself does cause serious and life-threatening effects in a certain percentage of patients. In the United States, virtually the only cases of polio which occur — several dozen per year — are caused by either the vaccine itself or infection from someone who recently received the vaccine. Based on my experience in China, I do not think Traditional Chinese Medicine alone is sufficient treatment for polio. Nevertheless, I also do not recommend this vaccine unless the child is going to travel to underdeveloped countries where polio is a present danger. If one decides to get this vaccine, one should ask for the killed vaccine rather than the live vaccine. The killed vaccine has a better safety record.

Measles, rubella & chickenpox

I do not recommend vaccinating for these diseases. In Asia, a childhood bout of any of these three diseases is not considered a bad thing. In Chinese medicine, these diseases are believed to be associated with so-called fetal toxins. It is said in Chinese pediatric books, "Because of fetal toxins accumulated, they are more susceptible to pox." Fetal toxins are toxins which are passed on to the baby at conception or developed in the womb. They lay dormant until they are provoked by some stimulating external pathogen. Then they are expressed to the surface of the body where they manifest as a rash or blisters. If these rashes or blisters are fully expressed and the body then heals correctly, the child is then better off for no longer harboring these fetal toxins. There are case

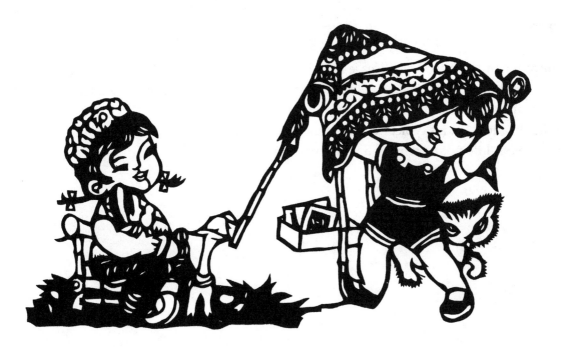

histories in the Chinese medical literature where chronic health problems which develop later in life are associated with incompletely expressed or expelled fetal toxins.

In addition, Chinese medicine does treat these three diseases very well. The main danger from measles is that it may develop into pneumonia. If treated correctly by Chinese medicine, this is very unlikely. However, if one does not choose to immunize their children against these three diseases, they should purposely expose their children to infection when they are still young. Measles and chickenpox tend to be worse for adults than for children, while German measles during pregnancy is associated with certain birth defects. In earlier times, people had measles and chickenpox parties so that their children would get these diseases, and there was wisdom behind that approach.

Mumps

Mumps is another infectious disease for which we can now immunize and which mostly strikes children. Chinese medicine treats mumps very well and this is not a serious disease unless it too is allowed to develop into pneumonia. It can, however, cause sterility in adults and is typically much more uncomfortable in adults than in children. Nonetheless, I do not recommend immunizing against it.

5
How Chinese Medicine Diagnoses Babies

Most of the treatments recommended in this book are for home care. They can be used as the first rung on that ladder of graduated responses we have talked about earlier. They can also be used in conjunction with other, professionally supplied treatments in order to make those treatments even more effective. In some cases, I have given the names of Chinese herbal formulas for particular patterns of specific diseases. I have mainly done this to give the reader an idea of how professionally applied Chinese medicine works. In order to apply Chinese herbal medicine correctly, one must be able to do a TCM pattern discrimination. Although that requires years of training in order to do it correctly, below I describe some of the types of things TCM practitioners look at and take into account when making a pattern discrimination on our little friends. This will enable parents to help collect the kinds of information the TCM practitioner will be looking for and will also give some hints to the parents about their child's condition.

Sun Si-miao (590-682), the most famous Chinese doctor of the Tang dynasty, said, "Better to treat 10 men than 1 woman; better to treat 10 women than 1 baby." What he meant by this was that, because women have menstrual cycles, there is more to take into account when diagnosing and treating them. Therefore, Sun felt it was harder to diagnose and treat women than men. Further, babies cannot talk. Therefore they cannot explain what they are feeling. Because of this, pediatrics has sometimes been jokingly referred to in Chinese medicine as specialization in mutes. Because he could not question his young patients the way he would adults, Sun felt that they were even more difficult to diagnose than women.

Happily, TCM gynecology and pediatrics has made great progress since the Tang dynasty, and I feel just the reverse of Sun Si-miao. If one understands the pivotal role of diet and indigestion in pediatrics, babies are actually much easier to treat than women. (And if one understands how to read the monthly report card of a woman's monthly cycle, women are much easier to diagnose than men who never tell you what is really going on anyway.) Therefore, I love to treat babies and do not find them all that difficult to diagnose. Essentially, what the Chinese doctor is trying to determine in most pediatric illnesses is whether the baby is abnormally hot or cold, whether their righteous or healthy qi is sufficient or insufficient, and whether there is some evil or unhealthy qi or substance which needs to be eliminated from the body. In order to make those determinations, the TCM practitioner uses four basic methods called the four examinations.

Looking

The first is looking. The practitioner looks at the baby's eyes and facial color, looks at the color of their hands and nails, looks at the vein at the base of the index finger, and looks at any particular area which is painful or diseased. Looking at the eyes tells the practitioner how serious the disease is. This is called inspecting the baby's spirit. If the eyes are clear and shining and the baby is aware and intelligent, then the disease is not all that serious and should respond to treatment without too much worry. If, on the other hand, the baby's eyes are dull, filmy, and lack awareness or consciousness, then the disease has become serious and great care needs to be taken, possibly including seeing a Western MD.

Next the practitioner looks at the color of the baby's skin. Is it redder than normal? If so, this suggests that there is some abnormal heat within the baby's body. Do they look sallow and pale? This suggests that there is not enough qi and blood for some reason.

Or do they look greenish blue? If so, they are probably either cold or in considerable pain. In particular, the practitioner will look at the vein at the root of the bridge of the nose between the two eyes. If a blue vein is visible here, this suggests that the baby's spleen, *i.e.*, their digestion, is weak, and the more prominent and visible this vein is, the weaker the spleen.

Then the practitioner will look at the vein at the base of the palmar side of the index finger. Traditionally, the left index finger was inspected in little boys and the right index finger in little girls. Depending upon the size, color, prominence, location, and shape of the vein here, the practitioner can tell whether the disease is hot or cold, excess or deficiency, how far it has progressed, and how dangerous the condition is. This inspection of the vein of children under six years of age is a diagnostic specialty within TCM pediatrics. It is one of the very important ways TCM pediatricians diagnose little children. This inspection tends to replace the feeling of the pulse at the radial artery, since children do not sit still well enough to make such pulse diagnosis really accurate. Therefore, the younger the child, the more important this inspection will be.

In addition, the TCM practitioner will also want to look at any place the child or the parent says they hurt or any location which is diseased. For instance, if there is a diaper rash, the practitioner will want to see that rash to determine what color red it is, how extensive it is, whether it is wet or dry, and whether the skin is broken or intact. Likewise, any other skin rash would be inspected in the same way. If a rash was very red, then this suggests pathological heat. If it is reddish purple, then the TCM practitioner may be thinking about TCM concepts such as toxins and/or blood stasis. If the rash is wet and weeping, this suggests pathologic dampness, while if there is pus production, this also suggests toxins.

Listening/smelling

In Chinese medicine, there is a single verb which translates as listening and smelling together. What the Chinese medical practitioner is listening for is the sound of any cough. Is it strong or weak? Is it wet or dry? Is it spasmodic? The practitioner also listens to the sound of breathing. Is it asthmatic and wheezing? Does it sounds phlegmy and obstructed? Further, the practitioner listens to the sound of the voice and the speech. Is the voice hoarse or raspy? Is the voice a normal loudness or very faint and weak? Can the child speak normally for their age? Are they delirious?

As for smelling, the practitioner smells the breath. This is very important for finding out if there is stagnant food in the stomach. If there is, the breath will tend to be sour and bad-smelling. If the breath is fresh and clean, then food stagnation is probably not the issue. Further, the practitioner will want to at least know from the parents how the stools smell. If they are very stinky, then there is probably heat and possibly food stagnation. If they are odorless, then perhaps the spleen is weak. Is the urine strong smelling? If it is, this again suggests heat. In actual practice, it is mostly the parents doing the smelling of the urine and stools and the practitioner questions the parents about this.

Feeling

When the child first comes in, the practitioner will usually pat the child's head and the side of their face. The parent may not know this, but the practitioner has already begun their diagnosis. By patting or stroking the head gently, the practitioner is seeing if the fontanelle has closed properly for the baby's age. By patting or stroking the baby's cheek, they can tell if the baby is hot or cold. They may then take the child's hands to play with, but while playing, they are also assessing whether the child is hot or cold. At some point in the examination, the practitioner will probably lie the child on their back and feel their abdomen. Is it too hot or cold? Is it too firm and distended or too slack and inform? The practitioner may or may not feel the baby's pulse at their wrist depending upon how old the child is, but the practitioner will want to feel any place the child or the parent says is affected by the complaint. For instance, if there is a sore throat (or even if there is not), the practitioner will want to feel the glands to see if they are swollen, hard, and/or tender to the touch.

Questioning

Although questioning the child itself is often not possible due to youngness of age, the practitioner will question the parent. They will want to know how the disease began, how long it has been going on, what are the symptoms, how is the appetite, the stools, urination, energy, mood, and sleep. What color is any phlegm? What treatments have already been tried and with what result? What does the child eat? What were they eating when they got ill? What else was happening when they got ill? Has the child had any fever? Do they seem to be running hot or cold, etc., etc.? Some of these questions are the same a Western MD might ask; others are specific to Chinese medicine. In all probability, the Chinese medical practitioner is going to be more interested in your child's diet, stools, appetite, and digestion than the Western physician.

The final TCM pattern discrimination or diagnosis will depend on the synthesis of information gathered by these four examinations. The TCM practitioner may or may not

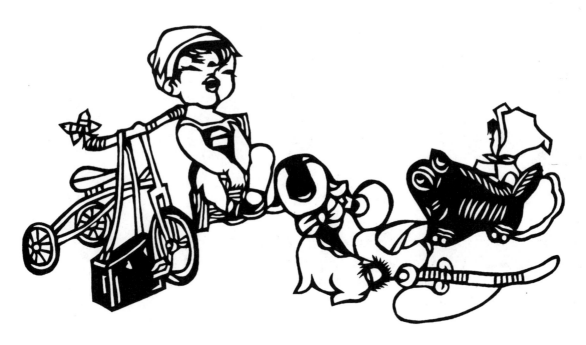

be interested in laboratory tests and cultures. But even if such tests have been done, the TCM pattern discrimination is not made on their basis. Rather, the TCM treatment should be based primarily on the TCM pattern of disharmony, and this is what makes TCM the safe and effective medicine it is.

When babies are first brought in to see the TCM practitioner, they may immediately recognize they are in a doctor's office, and they may start to cry, remembering the pokes and prods, jabs and shots they have received at Western MDs' offices. However, children soon learn that the TCM practitioner does not do any of that and that the visit is both gentle and kind. Therefore, children, by and large, love to go see their Chinese doctors. And I for one love to see them.

6
The Main Methods of Treating Children in Chinese Medicine

There are three main methods of professionally treating children in TCM besides adjusting their diets. It should be said at the outset that, without adjusting the diet, these three methods will not have a complete or lasting effect. The three main professional modalities for treating children in Chinese medicine are Chinese herbal medicine, Chinese pediatric massage, and acupuncture. Each of these methods have their own uses, advantages, and idiosyncracies. Some practitioners may practice all three of these modalities, while other practitioners may only practice one or two.

Chinese herbal medicine

Chinese medicine primarily means herbal medicine. Most TCM practitioners in China are herbal practitioners and the overwhelming majority of books and articles on Chinese medicine are about herbal medicine. In China, if one goes to a hospital or clinic and asks to see the pediatrician or pediatric ward, what one will see is the dispensing of Chinese herbal medicine. And if one picks up a book on Chinese pediatrics, the main treatment modality it will describe is Chinese herbal medicine.

Although this is called Chinese *herbal* medicine, in fact, not all the ingredients a TCM practitioner prescribes are "herbs." Herbs imply something from the vegetable kingdom, but a significant portion of the ingredients a Chinese doctor or TCM practitioner prescribes are from the animal and mineral kingdoms. When ingredients come from the vegetable kingdom, most of these ingredients are roots and barks with less of these ingredients being fruits and berries, twigs and stems, and leaves and flowers. Usually, anywhere between 4 and 20 ingredients are combined into a formula. It is rare that a professional TCM practitioner prescribes a single herb the way a Western folk herbalist might. These formulas are not just collections of all the ingredients the practitioner has heard are good for a particular problem. Rather, they are crafted together to act synergistically, each ingredient or couple of ingredients designed to accomplish a part of the overall process of restoring balance.

These Chinese herbal formulas are prescribed not for diseases but for the patient's individual pattern of disharmony. So, as we have seen above, it is not unusual for two patients with the same named disease to receive radically different Chinese herbal formulas. Because achieving and maintaining balance is an ever changing, fluid, and dynamic process, Chinese herbal formulas are changed every few days or every week or two. This is because people are always changing and Chinese herbal medicine treats people, not just diseases. Therefore, the process of doing Chinese herbal medicine usually requires close cooperation between the patient and practitioner.

There are a number of ways that Chinese herbal medicine can be dosed for children. There are pills, powders, alcohol tinctures, and so-called teas or decoctions. Many Chinese apothecaries in Chinatowns in the West carry a selection of ready-made patent medicines appropriate for children. A number of companies in Taiwan manufacture Chinese herbal extracts in powder form which are very high quality. Although these formulas are appropriate for children, because these powdered extracts do not dissolve as well as they might, they can be hard for children to take. Alcohol tinctures, primarily made in the West are easy to dose for children and easy to administer. If alcohol tinctures are used, parents should be sure to boil off the alcohol, since most children suffer from a degree of candidiasis which alcohol can aggravate. In order to evaporate off the alcohol, the dose should be added to some boiling water and allowed to sit for several minutes. The only problem with this is that then the child must take a larger quantity of liquid which may be difficult for the parent to get down.

In Chinese medicine, the tea or decoction is the standard method of administering Chinese herbal medicine, and Chinese pediatric texts overwhelmingly give decoctions as their treatment of choice. Some people, including some practitioners, say it is impossible to get an infant or toddler to drink a bitter decoction (and by adult standards, most Chinese decoctions are very bitter). However, it is my experience that children do not require the same amount of a prescription as an adult. Secondly, the amount they do need can be given in an eye-dropper. Many TCM practitioners when writing prescriptions for children reduce the dosages of the individual "herbs" but then direct that the parent make the tea with the same amount of water as they would for an adult formula. In our clinic, we write formulas for children with the same dosages as for adults, but then we give the child a reduced amount of the resulting decoction. For instance, we typically advise parents to boil one bag of herbs in two cups of water, until only one cup of liquid remains. That one cup is then reserved. The child is given 2 droppers two or more times per day depending upon how much of the decoction we think the child needs. A single bag of herbs dosed like this can last for five days to a week if it is refrigerated. If it is refrigerated, each individual dose should be warmed to at least body temperature.

I stress using an eye-dropper for administering decoctions to children because the child cannot spill when trying to bat it away the way they might a cup or a tablespoon. The dropper is inserted into their mouth and the bulb is squeezed. The herbs go in and down they go. The worst that can happen is for the baby to spit or drool some of the decoction back out, in which case, one can give a little more. Children's tastes are not the same as adults' and most of my little patients take Chinese herbs in this way without difficulty. If we were to taste their formula, we might wish to spit it out, but, surprisingly, many times children take the same brew without complaint. Some of these formulas can be flavored with a little sugar, but other formulas should not be. So that is something parents should ask their practitioner about. In general, the decoction should not be mixed in orange or other fruit juices, although there are a few exceptions to this.

When Chinese herbal medicines are used remedially with children, usually one stops treatment when the child is halfway better. This is one of the principles of treatment in Chinese pediatrics. This is because children typically respond to treatment very fast. The Chinese say this is because of their "pure" or "clean" organs and bowels. Usually, all children need to recover from the kinds of common conditions discussed in this book is a push in the right direction supported by proper diet and nursing. If one treats with herbal medicine for too long, the herbs themselves can actually create problems. On a number of occasions I have disregarded this advice and always with the universe giving me a good reminder. Typically what happens is that the child's major complaint, such as a cough or runny nose, gets better, but some other complaint crops up. When one goes to treat that secondary complaint, perhaps the original complaint comes back, and then one seesaws back and forth between these two. Whereas, if one simply stops administering the Chinese herbal medicine, all the complaints clear up without further to do.

Chinese pediatric massage

As mentioned above, there is a whole system of Chinese *xiao er tui na* or pediatric massage. Although I have never seen a pediatric acupuncture clinic in China, every hospital that has a massage ward has a pediatric massage clinic. Pediatric massage is a highly effective modality for treating all the commonly encountered pediatric diseases. It is gentle, safe, and without side effects. The child is not forced to take a pill or drink a bitter brew, nor are they poked by acupuncture needles. The younger the child is, the more effective pediatric massage is. Chinese pediatric massage is useful for treating children up to around the age of six.

Just as in Chinese herbal medicine, there are particular combinations of specific massage maneuvers for the rebalancing of particular patterns of disharmony. Therefore once again, two young patients with the same disease would not necessarily receive the same treatment, nor will the treatment be the same from treatment to treatment. Usually a Chinese pediatric massage treatment lasts 20-30 minutes. It is typically performed with the child clothed, although in the West with our central heating, the practitioner may prefer the child be in their diaper or underwear. If the condition is an acute one, the practitioner may want to do two treatments per day or at least one every day for a couple of days until the condition has markedly improved. If the condition is a chronic one, treatments are usually scheduled every other day. In fact, here in the West, that is Chinese remedial pediatric massage's main drawback — it needs to be done so frequently.

As discussed above, some pediatric massage techniques can be learned and practiced at home by parents. *Chinese Infant Massage Therapy* by Fan Ya-li and published by Blue Poppy Press is meant as a treatment manual for both professional practitioners *and* parents. It gives very simple TCM pattern diagnoses under each commonly encountered disease and each protocol is illustrated by pictures of every maneuver. My own personal suggestion is that, if one wants to use Chinese pediatric massage on their children, they should seek out a qualified professional practitioner who can 1) make the initial TCM pattern discrimination, 2) outline the maneuvers to be done each session, and 3) teach the parent how to do those maneuvers. Then armed with a book like Dr. Fan's, one will have a much greater chance of success.

Acupuncture & moxibustion

Acupuncture primarily refers to the insertion of very fine, sterile, stainless steel needles into certain spots on the body which have been proven for not less than 2,000 years to balance the qi and blood in the body in very specific ways. If one goes to an acupuncture clinic in a TCM hospital in China, one will see children being treated from time to time. However, to be frank, most children do not relish the idea of being stuck by a needle. Acupuncture needles do not hurt the way hypodermic needles do since they are much, much finer and nothing is injected into the body. Nonetheless, most children have already had one or more shots before coming to an acupuncturist's office and the prospect of another needle can easily reduce a child to a mass of squirming tears.

Acupuncturists have several ways of coping with this. First of all, some acupuncturists will only needle children on points on their back where the child cannot see what is going on. Secondly, most acupuncturists when needling children put the needles in, stimulate them for a moment or two, and then immediately take the needle right back out. In other words, needles are not usually left in place for 20-30 minutes the way they usually are in adults. Also, most acupuncturists will try to use less insertions than they would in an adult for the same condition. Remember, it is one of children's inherent characteristics that they transmit changes (both pathological *and* healing) more quickly and easily than adults.

But there are other ways to skin the proverbial cat, and most acupuncturists have other ways of treating our little friends. In the chapter on prevention, I mentioned the Japanese style of pediatric acupuncture referred to in the West as *shonishin*. This is the stimulation of acupuncture points on the outside of the body with various little tools, none of which penetrate the skin. These are mostly different kinds of brushes, scrapers, and rollers. This very gentle and benign method of stimulating acupuncture points can not only be used preventively but also remedially. Although I do not personally practice this system, I am told by practitioners who do that children respond to it very well *and that they love it.*

Some acupuncturists tape tiny magnets over the acupuncture points and stimulate the points that way. Magnetotherapy has been a part of Chinese medicine since at least the Tang dynasty (618-907). I have used this method myself with very good results. The points to be treated are selected and then the magnets are taped over the points with either their north or south poles facing the skin depending on whether or not one wants to tonify or sedate the point. These magnets can be left in place from overnight to several days at a time. Other acupuncturists stimulate points on children using various types of ionized pellets or medicinal herbs or pastes taped over the points.

Then there is laser acupuncture. This is a relatively new technique — new in comparison to the 2,000 plus year history of acupuncture. In laser acupuncture, a neon laser is used to stimulate the points to be treated. This is completely painless and yet effective. One can also use electrical stimulation of the points without inserting needles. In that case, blunt metal probes are held over the points or rubberized electrodes are taped over them. The practitioner can adjust the amount of current, *supplied by nothing more than a couple of flashlight batteries*, so that the child may or may not feel anything. Often, there is just the faintest little tingling sensation at each point. Electroacupuncture is also an effective method for treating children.

As with Chinese pediatric massage, usually more than a single treatment is necessary to cure most children's conditions. If the condition is acute, the practitioner might advise two treatments the first day. If the condition improves, then the child might receive one treatment per day for a couple or three days. As the condition continues to improve, treatments are spaced further out. Typically in the West, treatments for chronic conditions are given once per week with the exact number of treatments necessary for any given condition being very individualized.

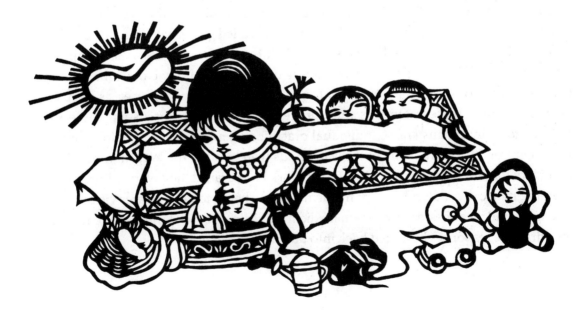

Moxibustion is the other half of what is simply referred to as acupuncture in the West. Moxibustion refers to the burning of a dried herb, Folium Artemisiae Argyii (*Ai Ye*) on, over, or near various acupuncture points or areas of the body. Moxibustion is mainly used in order to warm up areas of the body which are too cold or to add yang or warm qi to the body or specific organs of the body. Frequently, practitioners apply moxibustion by using a moxa roll. This is a big "cigar" of Artemisia or moxa which is lit and held near the acupoint or area which needs warming. Because warming also helps the qi and blood to move freely, moxibustion can also be used in cases where the intent is to promote more movement of the qi and blood. Moxibustion is often used to treat spleen and/or kidney deficiency conditions, and often practitioners teach parents how to do the moxibustion on their children at home. Usually such moxibustion is done once every day. The area which is moxaed becomes slightly red and warm to the touch but is not painful and does not, except in rare cases when this is intended by the practitioner, cause a blister or burn.

Other treatment methods

There are a number of other adjunctive or auxiliary treatment methods within the TCM armamentarium. These include cupping, scraping (called *gua sha* in Chinese), bleeding, various external applications, like plasters and ointments for skin diseases, the application of herbal medicines on particular acupuncture points or body parts, inhalants, eye, ear, and nose drops, etc. In the treatment sections under each of the diseases discussed below, various of these treatments appropriate for home use are discussed. These are not categorically exhaustive; so individual practitioners may have suggestions and treatments of their own. Many of these methods were used in the West in times past and were forgotten not because they didn't work but because they were eclipsed by the seeming magic of modern Western medicine. As we begin to get a clearer vision of the strengths and weaknesses of Western medicine, it is time some of these home remedies and first line responses be added back into our cultural repertoire.

7
Chinese Medicine & the Commonly Encountered Diseases of Children

The diseases discussed below are the most commonly encountered complaints among infants and young children. They have been arranged according to what is called a "longitudinal approach." This means that they appear in the order they are most likely to arise in terms of the age and development of the child. These are also the diseases which the parents can try to treat themselves with natural methods or for which Chinese medicine offers safe and effective treatments.

Neonatal jaundice

Many babies suffer from varying degrees of jaundice after birth. Jaundice means yellowing of the skin and possibly the whites of the eyes. Usually a small amount of neonatal jaundice is nothing to worry about. It can be treated by giving the baby water to drink and laying them in the sunlight. If, however, jaundice appears either within 24 hours of birth, is too dark a color, or persists too long after birth, Western doctors may want to treat this. Typically, Western medical treatment consists of keeping the baby in the hospital under so-called bilirubin lights and administering frequent feedings in order to help excrete the bilirubin.

Within Chinese medicine, the main treatments for this condition are Chinese herbal medicines. In order to make use of such medicines, the parents will have to take their baby to a professional practitioner of Chinese medicine. In general, the practitioner will decide which of two main patterns of neonatal jaundice your baby exhibits. If your baby has light but brightly colored yellow skin and eyes, deep yellow urine, and is warm to the touch and may be constipated, this is referred to as yang jaundice. If your baby has dull yellow colored skin and eyes, seems fatigued, has loose stools, and cold limbs, then this is yin jaundice.

In the case of yang jaundice, the treatment methods are to clear heat and eliminate dampness by promoting urination. In the case of yin jaundice, the treatment methods are to fortify or strengthen the spleen and warm yang while also promoting urination. The formula for treating yang jaundice is *Yin Chen Hao Tang* (Artemisia Capillaris Decoction) or something similar depending on the training, experience, and preference of the practitioner, while the formula for yin jaundice is *Yin Chen Li Zhong Tang* (Artemisia Capillaris Rectify the Center Decoction) or something similar. Whichever formula was prescribed would be boiled into a decoction or "tea" and given by eye-dropper several times per day. Generally, this condition is not treated with acupuncture, but rubbing of the abdomen to increase bowel movements is suggested.

Severe neonatal jaundice which does not respond to sunlight, water, rubbing of the abdomen, and/or Chinese herbal medicine does need to be treated by Western medicine, possibly including exchange blood transfusion. If left untreated, severe neonatal hyper-bilirubinemia may result in brain damage, seizures, and even death. Therefore, if the jaundice is severe, a Western MD should be consulted. Happily, this is the relatively rare exception rather than the rule.

Colic

Colic may occur anywhere from a few days to a few weeks after birth, and it may last from a couple of weeks to several months. Colic refers to gas pains in infants. The parent knows the baby is having such gas pains because the child cries and characteristically pumps their legs against their abdomen. The baby will want to be carried, held, and moved about. If and when the child passes gas, their crying diminishes or disappears. Usually the crying begins in the late afternoon or early evening and then may continue on through much of the night. In Chinese medicine, colic is traditionally described under the heading, night-crying. As the *Er Ke Zheng Zhi Xin Fa (Heart Methods of Patterns & Treatment in Pediatrics)* says:

> This disease mainly appears in newborns. During the day they are normal, but as they enter the night there is crying and restlessness. Each evening at the same time there is crying. If severe, this may continue throughout the night until dawn. Thus it is called night-crying.

This is a pretty good description of the timing and main symptoms of colic in young infants.

Colic can be very upsetting for the parents. Their baby is crying for some vague, undetermined reason. It is clear the baby is in pain, but the parent may not know why. Because the baby is crying and refuses to be put down or left alone, one or both parents may become exasperated and lose precious sleep. After a few nights of this, tempers can get short followed by guilty self-recriminations. In an attempt to pacify the baby, many parents try to assuage their child's crying by giving the baby the breast or a bottle. Unfortunately, this usually only makes the colic worse.

As with so many other pediatric complaints among infants and toddlers, colic is essentially a digestive complaint. In fact, it is *indigestion*. If, due to their inherently weak spleen or digestive power, the baby is not able to digest the milk or food that they are

69

given, it will accumulate and cause stagnation of the qi in the abdomen. Thus the abdomen becomes distended and the intestines become full of gas.

There are four main ways to prevent or eliminate colic according to Chinese medicine. The first and most important is to not overfeed the infant. Above we have discussed feeding on demand and the creation of food stagnation. Overfeeding jams the digestive mechanisms and leads to the accumulation of turbid qi and matter within the stomach and intestines. Therefore, feeding on schedule so as not to overstuff the infant's digestion and thus damage their already weak spleen, is the first and most important thing in preventing and treating colic. The fact that feeding should be on schedule and not on demand, according to Chinese medicine, is clearly and unambiguously stated in the following quote from *The English-Chinese Encyclopedia of Practical Traditional Chinese Medicine: Paediatrics* when speaking about the prevention of infantile dyspepsia or indigestion, *i.e.*, colic, "Regular diet (at fixed time and in fixed amount) and breast-feeding should be encouraged."

Secondly, one should rub the infant's abdomen daily as described in chapter four. Rubbing the abdomen from right to left following the direction of the large intestine helps to move the food through the digestive tract. This can be done preventively each day but may also be done remedially when and if colic occurs. When treating colic, that there is food stagnation is a given. However, in deciding what direction to rub the small circles, one needs to determine if the child is hot or cold. If they are hot, their face will become red when they cry, their hands and feet will be hot to the touch, and their cry will be loud and energetic. If they are cold, their face will be pale, a blue vein at the bridge of the nose will be visible, their hands and feet will be cold, and their cry will lack real force. If the child suffers from hot colic, then the small circles should be in the same direction as the large circles on the abdomen. If the child suffers from cold colic, meaning that their spleen is relatively weaker and needs strengthening beyond just moving stagnant food, then the small circles should go against the direction of the large circles. (For other infant massage techniques to treat this condition, see Fan Ya-li's *Chinese Infant Massage Therapy*.)

Third, the mother should avoid certain foods which tend to be gas-producing and colic-aggravating. According to Valerie Appleton, a midwife and acupuncturist, foods which the mother should avoid if her child has colic include the cabbage family (cabbage, broccoli, cauliflower, brussel sprouts, etc.), tomatoes, citrus fruits, garlic and onions, chocolate, and coffee. *The Merck Manual* fleshes out this list a bit by adding legumes, (*i.e.*, beans), rhubarb, peaches, and melons.

And fourth, if the colic does not respond to the above simple home remedies, one can treat it with Chinese herbal medicine. In that case, the practitioner will also determine whether the baby is more hot or more cold and will pick a Chinese herbal formula which either disperses accumulation and clears heat if the baby is too hot, or disperses accumulation and strengthens the spleen is the baby is too cold. If the colicky baby shows signs of neither hot nor cold, then the practitioner will simply disperse accumulation and harmonize the stomach. For instance, a formula called *Xiao Ru Wan* (Disperse Milk Pills) is often used for just food stagnation without hot or cold, another called *Bao He Wan* (Protect Harmony Pills) is frequently used for food stagnation and heat, and a modification of *Xiao Jian Zhong Tang* (Minor Fortify the Center Decoction) combined with *Li Zhong Tang* (Rectify the Center Decoction) is typically used for food stagnation and cold.

For colic due to food stagnation, one can take 60-90g of Mirabilitum (*Mang Xiao*) available from Chinese apothecaries or professional practitioners of Chinese herbal medicine and wrap this in a cotton bag. This is then placed over the navel and tied in place. If there is food stagnation and heat, one can make a tea out of parsley, hawthorne berries (available in Oriental specialty food shops and Chinese apothecaries under the name Fructus Crataegi [*Shan Zha*]), *daikon* radish, and orange peel. If there is colic due to food stagnation and internal cold due to spleen deficiency, then one can take 3 scallion stalks, 5 slices of fresh ginger, and 60-90g of wheat bran. Heat these together in a dry wok or fry pan and then wrap them in cotton cloth. While this bundle of herbs is still warm, "iron" around the abdomen with it.

In my experience, most Western babies with colic have food stagnation and heat. However, it is also common to see food stagnation, heat, and spleen weakness. In that case, one can still use the first three methods given above, but a professional practitioner will be necessary to either choose or to craft a Chinese herbal prescription which fits this slightly more complex pattern. *The Merck Manual* says that, "Parents should be assured that the colicky infant is basically healthy, that this behavior will cease in a few weeks, and that too much crying is not harmful." On the one hand that is good advice. On the other, Chinese medicine sees colic as one of the first steps in a potential series of health problems which can affect the constitutional balance and predispositions for one's entire life. If colic is treated at its root by using Chinese medicine both preventively and remedially, this can help prevent other health problems from occurring later on which also develop out of food stagnation and a weak spleen engendering dampness, phlegm, and pathological heat.

Vomiting of milk

Vomiting of milk refers to the baby's spitting up some milk after or during each feeding. According to Chinese medicine, this is also associated with the infant's inherently weak spleen and stomach. Just as colic is divided into several different patterns, vomiting in Chinese pediatrics can be subdivided into: food stagnation, spleen deficiency cold, spleen and stomach brewing of heat, liver invading the stomach, stomach yin deficiency, and fright and fear types. These patterns do not all appear in children of the same age. In infants, the two most commonly seen patterns are food stagnation and spleen deficiency cold types, and these two types are usually quite easy to distinguish.

In the food stagnation pattern of infantile vomiting, the baby vomits a sour, smelly vomitus of curdled milk which has lain in the child's stomach undigested. This often is referred to in the Chinese medical literature as vomiting undigested food eaten the night before. In addition, the baby will commonly have colic, gas, abdominal distention, and their breath does not smell sweet and clear like a baby's breath should. Rather it smells sour and fetid.

In the spleen deficiency cold pattern, the baby vomits back up the milk which has just been ingested. This vomitus looks just like the milk and does not have any bad smell. The hands and feet are usually cold, the face is pale, and there is typically a visible blue vein at the bridge of the nose. In addition, the vomiting is without force. The food wells back up but is not forcefully spit out. These signs show that the baby's spleen is too weak and cold to accept and digest the milk or other food. It is interesting to note that even the Western medical treatment handbook, *The Merck Manual*, says, "Excessive regurgitation may be due to overfeeding."

Both these types of infant vomiting are easy to treat. Rubbing the abdomen is especially good. Here one only has to distinguish whether to rub the small circles in the same direction as the large circles for food stagnation or to rub the small circles in the opposite direction as the large circles in the case of spleen deficiency. In addition, one can rub downward along the centerline of the abdomen a number of times for both types. One begins by rubbing from just under the ribs and ends at the baby's navel. In doing this maneuver, one should rub in one direction only — downward. Further, if the vomiting is of the spleen deficiency cold type, one can do the spinal pinch pull 3-5 times in order to strengthen the baby's righteous yang in general. Other Chinese pediatric massage maneuvers for both these types of infantile vomiting are described in *Chinese Pediatric Massage Therapy*.

As for feeding, in the case of food stagnation, the parent should feed the child less often or feed the child less every feeding. This allows the body to deal with the accumulated superabundance which the child has not already been able to digest. A simple home remedy consists of 25g of grated fresh ginger and 50g of dried orange peel made into a tea. This can then be given to the child through a bottle instead of, or before breast-feeding.

In the case of spleen vacuity cold, it is especially important to feed the child small, frequent, easily digestible foods. Here one should remember the concept of 100° soup. The spleen deficiency child should not be given anything dry and hard to digest, nor should they be given anything chilled or raw. All their food should be cooked and served warm. As for spices, a little dry ginger powder, some cardamon powder, or a little cinnamon powder can help strengthen the spleen and warm deficiency cold. A simple home remedy for this type of vomiting is to make a tea out of 5 black dates (available from Oriental specialty food stores or Chinese apothecaries) and a few whole cloves. Crush the cloves and boil with the dates in water. Another simple Chinese herbal home remedy for this type of children's vomiting is to make a tea out of 4g of fresh ginger and 8g of dried orange peel. (This latter remedy is also good for cough with excessive damp phlegm.)

In the same way, there are different Chinese herbal formulas for both of these two patterns. Modified *Bao He Wan* (Protecting Harmony Pills) is the usual guiding formula for food stagnation vomiting, while modified *Li Zhong Tang* (Rectify the Center Decoction) is the common guiding formula for spleen deficiency cold vomiting.

Vomiting due to fear and fright is also seen in infants. It is said in Chinese pediatrics, "Because of cowardly spirit qi, they easily become emotionally upset." Children with this pattern seem to be simply constitutionally high-strung and easily scared. In premodern times, Chinese doctors talked about the negative effects of fright encountered in the womb. However, I have not been able to confirm any such instances of *in utero* trauma in my young patients who have exhibited this pattern.

The clinical manifestations of this pattern are vomiting of clear fluids, a pale but bluish green complexion, restlessness, sudden jerking movements of the body during sleep, disturbed sleep, and frequent spells of crying as if frightened for some reason. Mostly this pattern of pediatric vomiting should be treated with Chinese herbal medicine, Chinese infant massage, or some sort of "acupuncture" stimulation. The treatment principles are to level the liver and extinguish wind, downbear counterflow and stop vomiting. The diet should be designed to strengthen the spleen, while the parents should give the child a lot of emotional assurance of safety, care, and love. Perhaps the child had a traumatic past life, but at least their present parents can convey through their love and care that the child is safe and wanted in their new family.

Spleen and stomach brewing heat vomiting is more commonly met with in a somewhat older toddler or young child. Usually these children have begun eating solid foods and have developed a taste for greasy foods, such as chips, peanut butter, hot dogs and hamburgers, etc. Such greasy, fried, fatty foods are, according to Chinese dietary therapy, inherently hot but also hard to digest. If the child eats too much of this sort of food, it may sit in the stomach and smolder and brew into a type of damp heat. This child also may have bad breath, but we know that the child's TCM pattern is one of heat because the vomiting has more force and may even be projectile. Typically, the child's face is red and their hands and feet are hot. Their urine is darkish, their stools may be either constipated and hard or loose, explosive, smelly, and burn around the anus. The vomitus itself also smells fetid.

Spleen and stomach brewing heat should first be treated by identifying the offending foods. These then should be removed from the child's diet. In my experience, children with this pattern also eat a lot of sugar which, according to Chinese medicine, is also very dampening. Once the offending foods have been removed, it is wise to feed the child what the Chinese call a clear, bland diet for several days. This means a vegetarian diet consisting of rice porridge and steamed and mashed vegetables without any fat, grease, or hot spices. Besides modifying the child's diet, one can also rub the abdomen, again with small circles in the direction of the large circles, and rub down the midline of the baby's abdomen above the navel. The commonly used Chinese herbal formula for this type of pediatric vomiting is called modified *Huo Po Huang Lian Tang* (Agastaches, Magnolia & Coptis Decoction). This formula contains ingredients to clear heat from the spleen and stomach, eliminate dampness, and direct the upwardly counterflowing qi, manifesting as vomiting, back downward. A simple home remedy is to make a "tea" out of a little umeboshi paste (available at health food stores), grated ginger, and some kudzu root power (also available at health food stores).

Liver invading the stomach vomiting is also typically seen in an older child. In many ways, it is the same or similar pattern as vomiting due to fear and fright, but in an older child. Children with this pattern are usually high-strung and high-spirited. Because of this, they often become angry, and this anger may manifest as either outbursts or repression. Anger is the emotion associated with the liver. As long as the child's qi is not thwarted, the liver's qi is able to flow smoothly and without inhibition. But if this qi is repressed or thwarted, the liver may become depressed. This means that the qi of the liver stagnates and accumulates. Eventually this stagnant and accumulated qi has to go somewhere and commonly it vents itself on the stomach and/or spleen. This is also what "venting one's spleen" originally meant in English. Because the liver qi invades or attacks the stomach qi, the stomach qi counterflows upward and this counterflow manifests itself as vomiting.

The main sign of this pattern of pediatric vomiting is vomiting after some emotional upset. The child may appear angry or withdrawn. Usually they will have a red face when vomiting, and, in particular, the vomitus will mostly consist of sour water or bile. The first measure to be taken in treating this pattern of vomiting is to identify the cause and remedy the situation at its source. That does not mean that the parents should capitulate to the child's every wish and whim. Rather, the child needs to be taught better coping skills for dealing with anger and frustration. They should be encouraged to talk things out. They may not like a particular situation, but "everything" is not "always" a disaster.

In terms of pediatric massage, the parent should first massage the child's head and neck. Using your two thumbs, gently and soothingly draw the thumbs across the child's forehead from the middle out toward the temples. Massage the child's temples in a circular motion, and massage the back of the child's neck under the base of their skull. These are all the same places adults store stress and tension. In Chinese pediatric massage, these maneuvers are believed to calm the child's spirit, which, in this pattern, is vitally important. Then one can go on to massaging the abdomen with small circles going in the same direction as the large circles and then the pushing down the center of the abdomen.

A very good Chinese herbal formula for this pattern of pediatric vomiting is *Jie Gan Jian* (Resolve the Liver Decoction). It includes ingredients which soften and harmonize the liver, downbear upward counterflow, regulate the qi, and specifically stop vomiting. *Shonishin* acupuncture can also be a good choice for treating this pattern.

Stomach yin deficiency vomiting describes a child who has vomited so much or for so long that they have developed dry heaves. Therefore, this pattern typically describes a chronic condition, not an episodic or acute one. Chinese medicine is particularly adept at identifying healthy energies within the body that have become depleted and then restoring them with herbal supplementation. In fact, this condition is best treated by Chinese herbal medicine. The commonly used formula is modified *Sha Shen Mai Dong Tang* (Glehnia & Ophiopogon Decoction). This formula contains within it ingredients that nourish stomach yin and help generate body fluids as well as to stop vomiting. Cooked applesauce or cooked mashed pears can be useful foods to help the child recuperate from this pattern.

If there is repeated projectile vomiting, meaning that the vomit launches out of the child's mouth with great force and carries for some distance, this may signal a more serious condition, such as pyloric stenosis or gastroesophageal reflux. I have treated several cases of projectile vomiting in toddlers whose pattern was damp heat brewing in the spleen and stomach due to eating too many greasy, fatty foods. However, if dietary changes and some Chinese herbal medicine do not bring projectile vomiting quickly to an end, the child should be taken to see a Western MD.

Diarrhea

Diarrhea in infants and children is usually divided into four main patterns. The first is stagnant food diarrhea. This is due to overfeeding or overeating. The food is not digested but rather accumulates and putrefies within the stomach and intestines. Its symptoms are nausea, bad breath, abdominal distention, crying from pain before the movement and stopping of crying after the diarrhea, putrid, foul-smelling stools or sour-smelling stools, undigested food in the stools, having diarrhea 5-6 times each day and even up to 10 times or more, a thick, slimy tongue coating which may be slightly yellowish, and a slippery pulse. In young infants, the key signs are the bad breath, the foul-smelling stools with undigested food, and an engorged, purplish vein at the base of the index finger.

The treatment principles are to disperse food and lead away stagnation. Professional practitioners will probably prescribe a formula similar to *Bao He Wan* (Protecting Harmony Pills) with various modifications. Feeding should be reduced but warm, clear water should be given.

Chinese infant massage of the belly is very helpful. In this case, one wants to do circular rubbing with clockwise circles within the larger circle in order to promote the expulsion of the stagnant food in the intestines.

The second pattern of pediatric diarrhea is wind cold. This is an external invasion pattern due to having caught a cold. Its symptoms are watery stools with a lot of froth or foam and which are pale in color and only smell very slightly. There is abdominal pain and intestinal noises or borborygmus. In addition, there is accompanying fever, stuffy nose, runny nose, slight cough, lack of appetite, no increased thirst, a slimy, white tongue coating, and a soggy pulse. The treatment principles for this type of diarrhea are to course wind, scatter cold, and transform dampness. One representative formula for this type of pattern is *Huo Xiang Zheng Qi San* (Agastaches Correct the Qi Powder) with modifications. However, I do not see much of this kind of diarrhea in my patient population.

The third pattern of pediatric diarrhea is damp heat. Its symptoms are fever, thirst, abdominal pain accompanying diarrhea, up to 20 movements per day which are greenish or yellow in color and smell foul, redness, heat, and burning around the anus, a slimy, yellow tongue coating, and a slippery, rapid pulse. In this case, the stools are putrid but there is not particularly bad breath. In addition, the color of the stools and the redness and irritation around the anus are all indications of damp heat. The treatment principles are to clear heat and disinhibit dampness. One commonly prescribed formula for this type of damp heat diarrhea is *Ge Gen Qin Lian Tang* (Pueraria, Scutellaria & Coptis Decoction) with various additions and subtractions depending on the case. In such patterns, it is important to avoid all greasy, fatty foods and anything hot and spicy. Chinese pediatric massage is not so effective, but Chinese herbal medicine for this pattern is very effective.

The fourth pattern of pediatric diarrhea is spleen deficiency. This is due to the spleen being too weak to digest foods and liquids properly. Thus the pure and impure of foods and liquids are not separated but rather pour downward undigested. The symptoms of this type of diarrhea are chronic diarrhea or sometimes diarrhea and sometimes vomiting, loose, watery stools, undigested food or milk in the stools, diarrhea after eating and several times a day, poor appetite, fatigue, lack of strength, a pale or yellow face and pale lips, a blue vein at the root of the nose, cold limbs, a pale tongue with a thin, slimy coating, and a deep, forceless pulse. The treatment principles are to fortify the spleen and warm the middle. *Qi Wei Bai Zhu San* (Seven Flavors Atractylodes Powder) with modifications would be a typically prescribed Chinese herbal formula.

With this last type of diarrhea, proper diet is very important. This means a diet of cooked, warm foods, no frozen, chilled, or iced foods or liquids, no (or very few) raw foods, a clear, bland diet, and little or no sugar. Spinal pinch pull up the spine several times a day can strengthen the spleen and generally strengthen the qi. Acupuncturists or professional practitioners of Chinese medicine may want to teach the parents how to do moxibustion on certain points. For instance, a slice of ginger may be placed on the navel and then Artemsia Argyium or moxa may be burnt over that daily in order to strengthen the digestion. In addition, some warming, spleen-strengthening spices may be added to the food, such as cardamom, fennel, dry ginger powder, a little cinnamon, some cloves, and/or a little nutmeg. Practitioners of Chinese medicine may also recommend making a porridge out of any of several, very bland-tasting, spleen-strengthening Chinese herbs which can be ground into powder and then cooked into a gruel. These include Radix Dioscoreae Oppositae (*Shan Yao*), Sclerotium Poriae Cocos (*Fu Ling*), Semen Coicis Lachryma-jobi (*Yi Yi Ren*), and Semen Dolichoris Lablab (*Bai Bian Dou*).

Another remedy for this type of diarrhea is to pound several cloves of garlic and wrap them in clean cotton gauze. Then tie this herbal compress directly over the navel. And yet another home herbal remedy for this type of deficiency diarrhea is to powder some cloves and cinnamon bark, place this powder in the child's navel, and then hold in place with an adhesive plaster. Children with diarrhea in general and with this pattern of diarrhea in particular should not be allowed to eat honey.

According to Western medicine, persistent diarrhea in infants may be due to an adverse reaction to wheat gluten, insufficiency in pancreatic enzymes, sugar malabsorption, and food allergies. Pancreatic enzymes are very much related to the Chinese idea of spleen function, some Western authors saying the Chinese medical concept of the spleen should be called the spleen-pancreas. The clear, bland diet of Chinese medicine for babies is mostly a wheat-free diet. Sugar malabsorption and food allergies are also addressed by the clear, bland diet and Chinese herbal medicine. If there is sudden onset of vomiting, bloody stools, fever, loss of appetite, and listlessness, this suggests dysentery or infectious diarrhea. Even this can be treated with Chinese herbal medicine. However, if Chinese medicine does not bring this quickly to a halt, the baby should see a Western MD.

Diaper rash

Diaper rash refers to chapping and chafing of the skin due to wet diapers. In Chinese, this is referred to as *yan kao chuang*, "neglected tailbone sores." It was described in the Chinese medical literature as early as 610 AD. In general, this condition is described as a damp heat pattern. It is a heat pattern because the skin is red in color and hot to the touch. It is damp because there may be small water blisters, wet-looking sores, or the condition is aggravated on exposure to dampness, *i.e.*, the soaking dampness of an unchanged diaper. Chinese medicine primarily treats diaper rash with various external applications.

If your child develops diaper rash, you probably need to change their diaper more often. Once the rash has occurred, one should leave off the diaper altogether in order to let the rash dry out. In addition, there are several powders that can be dusted on which can be gotten from a Chinese herbalist or apothecary. The first is Terra Flava Usta (*Fu Long Gan*). This is a fine powder made from the inside of clay stoves in China. The other is a combination of Talcum (*Hua Shi*) and Pulvis Indigonis (*Qing Dai*). These two ingredients are powdered finely and mixed together at a ratio of 5 parts Talcum to 1 part Indigo. Indigo is a very powerful antifungal, antibacterial herb in Chinese medicine. If the skin is dry, scaly, and chapped rather than ulcerated and wet, one can apply roasted sesame seed oil. Roasted sesame seed oil is available from Oriental specialty food shops and health food stores.

For really severe diaper rash, Chinese medical practitioners can prescribe herbal washes and stronger ointments than just roasted sesame seed oil.

In Western medicine, diaper rash is usually seen as a yeast infection or candidiasis. Whenever there is candidiasis, a clear, bland diet should be instituted. In a breast-fed baby, this means that the mother should go on a clear, bland diet. For more information on a clear, bland diet and candidiasis, the reader may see my *Arisal of the Clear: A Simple Guide to Healthy Eating According to Traditional Chinese Medicine* from Blue Poppy Press.

Prickly heat

Prickly heat is also called miliaria. It is a commonly seen skin ailment in the summertime caused by inadequate perspiration in unduly hot weather. It begins with small little papules or bumps or even tiny little blisters with a red base, each of which has distinct borders but which may blur together gradually into a patch. The skin feels hot to the touch and there is an itchy sensation.

One remedy for prickly heat besides removing tight or hot garments and bathing frequently is to rub fresh cucumber slices over the affected area.

Cradle cap

Cradle cap refers to seborrheic dermatitis in infants. It may develop within the first month of life and is characterized by a thick, yellow, crust on the scalp. If more severe, there can also be cracking and yellow scaling behind the ears and red papules on the face. Many children with cradle cap are also prone to diaper rash, and this fact gives a hint as to its cause and treatment. As we have seen above, diaper rash is due to a damp heat condition. According to Chinese medicine, children as well as adults typically exhibit a single, overall pattern. That pattern may be complex and multifaceted, but that is the difference between a TCM pattern and a disease. The pattern takes into account all the person's signs and symptoms and tries to recognize the total pattern as a single *gestalt*.

If one analyses the lesions on the top of the head, what one sees in cradle cap is a thick, dry, yellow crust. According to the logic of TCM, such dry, crusty skin lesions suggest a dry disease mechanism. However, if there is damp heat smoldering and brewing within the child, the heat component typically wafts upward because heat inherently rises. This heat then dries out the upper regions of the body even though its origin is a damp heat below. Thus it is not at all uncommon in either children or adults to see damp heat symptoms below and dry heat symptoms above, and, if one understands this aspect of damp heat, one can recognize these two seemingly contradictory manifestations as parts of the same pattern.

Therefore, the treatment of cradle cap should be two pronged. On the one hand, the child may be given some Chinese herbal medicine designed to clear heat and eliminate dampness. What Chinese herbs must depend on the signs and symptoms and the severity of the condition. Because there are a number of possibilities, this determination needs to be left up to a professional practitioner of Chinese medicine. Usually the formula will be a combination of heat-clearing, dampness-eliminating medicinals and spleen-strengthening, digestion-improving ingredients.

Locally, the parent can massage a small amount of roasted sesame seed oil into the lesion each night. This is left on during sleep and then shampooed out. If the child is eating solid foods, they should not be fed any sugar or sweets, nor should they be allowed to drink sweet fruit juices. It is important to note that a bottle of fruit juice can have as much or more sugar as a candy bar.

According to Western medicine, cradle cap is associated with genetic and climactic factors. According to TCM theory, the propensity towards cradle cap is usually developed while the child is in the womb. Commonly, mothers during pregnancy have eaten too many sugars and sweets and/or greasy, spicy, fatty, "hot foods." These types of foods lead to a damp heat condition in the mother which is then passed on to the child. Therefore, eating a nutritious, clear, bland diet during pregnancy is one way to prevent this condition. Although a clear, bland diet is *mainly* a vegetarian diet, it may contain a small, regular amount of animal protein as long as that animal protein is not overeaten or too greasy and fatty. In addition, it is also important for breast-feeding mothers of babies with cradle cap to eat a clear, bland diet.

Oral thrush

Oral thrush refers to an overgrowth of fungus in the mouth. It typically causes creamy or milky patches on the tongue or insides of the mouth with inflammation of the underlying tissue. It is also referred to as oral candidiasis. In Chinese pediatrics, there are several textbook patterns corresponding to oral thrush. The two most important of these are: 1) spleen/stomach accumulation and heat and, 2) deficiency heat floating upward. However, in actual clinical practice, most cases do not divide so neatly into excess and deficiency patterns. In fact, in my experience, most cases of pediatric thrush are a combination of damp heat in the stomach *with* spleen deficiency. In such cases, the spleen deficiency is due to the spleen's inherent weakness in infants aggravated by faulty feeding or poor diet. The damp heat is due to over-feeding or faulty diet.

When there is a combination of factors causing oral thrush in infants and toddlers, as there most often is, the accompanying signs and symptoms are also a mixture of excess and deficiency. For instance, the lesions are recurring and do not heal, the appetite is not good, the facial complexion is a sallow yellow, and the stools are loose. Therefore, the treatment principles are to supplement the center and boost the qi, suppress and downbear yin fire using a combination of sweet, warm and bitter, cold ingredients. Based on these principles, a modified version of *Bu Zhong Yi Qi Tang* (Supplement the Center & Boost the Qi Decoction) may be prescribed which also contains several ingredients known to be antifungal. In addition, it is usually a good idea to use a Chinese herbal powder blown into the mouth and directly onto the oral lesions. In that case, the powdered herbs applied directly to the thrush itself are mostly antifungals, while the internal medication is a combination of spleen-strengthening and antifungal herbs.

Because the child has candidiasis, it is usually helpful and important for the mother to go on a clear, bland, anti-candidal, or hypoallergenic diet while the baby is being treated. This is described in some detail below under pediatric allergies. If the mother suffers from polysystemic chronic candidiasis (PSCC), then it is not uncommon for the mother to develop cracked nipples at the same time as the child has oral candidiasis. In that case, besides the mother adopting a clear, bland, yeast-free, sugar-free diet, she should also apply Chinese antifungal medicinals to her cracked nipples. If there is a lot of oozing from the cracks, then a powdered medicine is made from Radix Angelicae Dahuricae (*Bai Zhi*), mixed with breast milk, and applied to the nipples. If the nipples are cracked, dry, and chapped but not oozing or suppurating, then a Chinese herbal salve, such as *Qing Dai Gao* (Indigo Ointment) can be used between feedings.

Because polysystemic chronic candidiasis can play a role in so many other chronic conditions, I believe it is important to treat fungal conditions such as thrush quickly and comprehensively whenever they appear. For me, this always means taking into account the diet as well as any other remedial treatment. This means that both the baby and the breast-feeding mother should be eating a clear, bland diet. What a clear, bland diet means for an infant is either breast milk or, if they are on formula, a formula without added sugar. If they are already on solid foods, they should not be given foods with added sugar or fruits and fruit juices. The best food for an infant other than breast milk is a dilute soup made out of white rice, rice being the most hypoallergenic and easy to digest grain.

Teething

Teething is not listed as a disease in Chinese pediatric books. Rather, teething is a normal physiological event in the process of the child's maturation. However, teething may be accompanied by pain and even fever. In Chinese medicine, physiological changes or transformations are warm transformations. The term for maturation in Chinese is *cheng shu*. The word *cheng* means to become, while the word *shu* means to ripen but also to cook. Its radical is the fire radical implying cooking. As parents know, children do not develop steadily at a single pace. Development comes in fits and starts. There are periods of recuperation and preparation and then periods of rapid growth and change. In Chinese medicine, such periods of accelerated growth and change are associated with extra heat in the body, and this extra heat may cause transient fever. This is referred to as *bian zheng*, change and steaming.

As we will see below, there are a number of ways parents can help relieve their child's fever and one or more of these can be used if fever accompanies teething. If the fever which often is associated with teething is not too high and if the child is not in great pain or discomfort, it does not necessarily require treatment. However, I have found in my practice that often a few doses of a very simple Chinese herbal formula called *Suan Zao Ren Tang* (Zizyphus Spinosae Decoction) can reduce the fever and the fretfulness of teething. Your local practitioner can decide whether or not this is appropriate for your particular child. As we will also see below, sometimes this change and fever may set off or aggravate an ear infection and these most definitely can and should be treated by Chinese herbal medicine.

Fever

Fever may occur in infants and toddlers either all by itself or in combination with some other problem such as a cold or earache. Often times, fever is the main way a parent knows their child is ill, and children's fevers tend to be higher than adults and, therefore, more frightening. In Chinese medicine, fevers are divided into two broad categories of patterns. There are patterns associated with invasion of the exterior by external pathogens and there are patterns referred to as internal damage patterns. The first group of patterns (invasion of the exterior by external pathogens) are associated with recent onset, acute conditions, while the second group of patterns (internal damage) are associated with chronic conditions.

There are four external invasion patterns of fever in TCM pediatrics. They are wind cold, wind heat, warm heat, and damp heat, each of which has its own signs and symptoms, treatment principles, and treatment plans. Wind cold is characterized by a stuffy nose, runny nose, cough, aversion to cold, fever, headache, no sweating, muscular aches and pains, a thin, white tongue coating, and a floating pulse. In this case, the treatment principles are to course wind and scatter cold and to use acrid, warm medicinals to resolve the exterior. A common Chinese herbal formula fitting this bill would be *Jing Fang Bai Du San* (Schizonepeta & Ledebouriella Vanquish Toxins Powder) with various modifications.

If the child has a wind heat pattern, they will typically display a stuffy nose, cough, slight aversion to cold, fever, headache, slight perspiration, a red, painful throat, a thin, white or slightly yellow tongue coating, and a floating, rapid pulse. In this case the treatment principles are to course wind and clear heat and use acrid, cool medicinals to resolve the exterior. A commonly used formula for this pattern of pediatric fever is *Sang Ju Yin* (Morus & Chrysanthemum Drink) or *Yin Qiao San* (Lonicera & Forsythia Powder) with modifications depending upon the exact signs and symptoms of each child. A simple Chinese herbal home remedy for a wind heat pattern of fever is to boil some marjoram in water to make into a "tea", then drink this to induce perspiration. Marjoram is acrid and cool and thus resolves the exterior while clearing heat.

In the warm heat pattern, there is a high fever which does not abate, annoying or upsetting thirst, definite perspiration, a red tongue with a dry, yellow coating, and a slippery, rapid pulse. In this case, warm hot pathogens have entered the body more deeply than in the two previous patterns. The treatment principles are to clear heat and nourish fluids, and a representative formula your practitioner might prescribe would be *Lian Qiao San* (Lonicera & Forsythia Powder) plus *Shi Gao Zhi Mu Tang* (Gypsum & Fibrosum Decoction) with various additions and subtractions to meet your child's individual needs.

And if the child is suffering with a damp heat pattern, then there is a fever which is not very high, fullness or tightness in the head, lack of strength in the four limbs, a tight or heavy feeling in the chest, nausea, a dry mouth but only scanty drinking, a bland taste in the mouth, poor appetite, reddish, *i.e.,* darkish urine, possible loose stools, a thick, slimy, white tongue coating, and a soggy, rapid pulse. The treatment principles are to clear heat and disinhibit dampness using medicinals which are penetratingly aromatic and which transform turbidity. *Huo Po Xia Ling Tang* (Agastaches, Magnolia, Pinellia & Poria Decoction) plus *San Ren Tang* (Three Seeds Decoction) with modifications is one combination which fills this bill.

In all four of these patterns, one should not try to bring down the fever by immersing the child or bathing the child in cold water. Since these are primarily external invasion patterns, bathing the child will only close the pores of the skin, while the Chinese medical practitioner is trying to do just the opposite — to open the pores and allow the pathogens to leave the body.

One can use the repeated massage down the spine to try to lower the fever in all these cases. One can also scrape the shoulders and back of the neck with a Chinese soup spoon until the skin of the upper back and neck have turned red. This is called *gua sha* and is one way of opening or resolving the exterior to allow for the outward dissipation of the heat.

For the wind heat, warm heat, and damp heat types of fever, drinking the juice of 2-3 freshly mashed star fruits or carambola 2-3 times per day is a specific remedy in Chinese dietary therapy for reducing fever. However, these fruits are by nature cold and should not be used in either the wind cold type of fever or the qi and blood deficiency fever described below.

Another way of bringing down fever in the three heat patterns above is to prick certain acupuncture points to allow one or two drops to escape. This should be done by a licensed acupuncturist or otherwise professionally qualified practitioner of Chinese medicine.

There are two so-called internal damage patterns of fever in TCM pediatrics. Although the word damage may sound dangerous, the use of this word is just technical jargon and does not imply a dangerous or serious condition. What it means is that a disease has dragged on for some time and has damaged one of the body's righteous energies or substances, and it is this damage of the righteous energy which is making the case hard to heal. These two internal damage conditions are not commonly seen in outpatient practice. Children who have these patterns are ill with some disease, such as rheumatoid arthritis, pertussis, or some other chronic condition for which they are probably already under medical care. These patterns are not associated with high fevers which come out of nowhere in the middle of the night.

The first internal damage fever pattern is called yin deficiency, internal heat pattern. Its symptoms are tidal fever (meaning a fever which returns at intervals, such as every evening), night sweats, flushed cheeks, a vexed spirit (meaning an irritated, easily annoyed, restless spirit), a dry cough with little phlegm, a dry throat, dry lips, thirst, short, reddish (*i.e.*, darker than normal) urine, dry stools, a red tongue with a scanty coating or a possibly geographic, peeling tongue coating, and a fine, rapid pulse. The treatment principles are to nourish yin and clear heat, moisten dryness and generate fluids. Professional practitioners of Chinese medicine typically prescribe formulas such as *Qin Jiao Bie Jia San* (Gentiana Macrophylla & Carapax Amydae Powder) combined with *Sha Shen Mai Dong Tang* (Glehnia & Ophiopogon Decoction) with various modifications. Children with this kind of deficient, dry, hot condition should be given pear sauce and applesauce and maybe even a little warm milk and sugar.

The second internal damage pattern of fever is called qi and blood dual deficiency pattern. Its symptoms are a low-grade fever which is aggravated by or comes on when there is fatigue, spontaneous perspiration or sweating on slight exertion, scanty appetite, loose stools, lassitude of the spirit (meaning a listless, colorless affect and facial complexion), fatigue, a lusterless facial complexion and pale lips, a weak voice or disinclination to speak, a pale tongue with a white coating, and a fine, soft pulse. The treatment principles are to fortify or strengthen the spleen and boost the qi while using warm and sweet medicinals to eliminate heat. Professional practitioners commonly prescribe formulas such as *Yi Gong San* (Strange Effect Powder) combined with *Bu Zhong Yi Qi Tang* (Supplement the Center & Boost the Qi Decoction) with various modifications. Children with this pattern should be fed a warm, nutritious, clear bland diet, and they should be treated with the spinal pinch-pull manuever of Chinese pediatric massage every day to strengthen their constitution.

Chinese medicine really excels at treating the two above kinds of deficiency patterns. These are the kinds of patterns that Western medicine typically does not treat very well. Antibiotics usually do not achieve any effect in these types of patterns because the issue is not the presence of pathogens or germs but the run-down strength of the body's immunity. Chinese herbal medicine is extremely effective for promoting the health of the body and for strengthening the immunity. Therefore, parents of children suffering from chronic conditions accompanied by either recurrent or low-grade fevers should definitely give Chinese herbal medicine a try.

Ear infections

Ear infections are one of the most common pediatric complaints in the West. These typically occur for the first time around the time of first teething. This is also right around the time that many parents introduce solid foods for the first time. Usually, the parent first notices that the child is crying as if in pain. Secondarily, they may see that the child is pulling on or batting their ear. If one of these two things don't get the parent's attention, then a fever accompanying these other two surely does. If taken to a Western MD, the standard treatment is antibiotics. This does usually put an end to the current acute condition. But all too often, the child develops another earache soon after the course of antibiotics is over. Again the child is put on antibiotics and again, when they are over, the earache comes back. If this continues enough times, the parents will be advised to have tubes surgically implanted in the child's eardrum to allow drainage and prevent rupture with subsequent possible hearing loss. As a clinician, I can't tell you how many times I have heard this story.

When I was studying pediatrics in China, several of my teachers asked one day what were the most commonly seen pediatric conditions in the United States. I unhesitatingly answered ear infections. The good doctors conferred for a moment amongst themselves and then turned to me to say that ear infections were not a very big problem in China. In fact, of the dozen or so Chinese pediatric texts I consulted when putting together this book, only one even had a section on ear infections! Some Western doctors tell parents that infants and toddlers are prone to ear infections because of the short distance between the nasal cavity and the eustachian canals which lead to the inner ear. Therefore, the thinking goes, germs can easily travel from the nose to the ear in the very young. Well, I cannot believe that Chinese babies' eustachian canals are located that much further from the nasal cavity than Western babies'. So clearly something else must be at work in Western babies.

In Chinese medicine when dealing with ear infections in adults, there are a number of patterns of disharmony, each with their own treatment principles and methods. However, in toddlers and young children, the situation is very much simplified. According to Chinese medicine, there is an internal pathway or connection between the stomach and intestines and the inner ear. If stagnant food accumulates in the stomach and intestines, this may give rise to transformative heat as described above. If there is fever associated with teething, this heat and the heat associated with the stagnant food may aggravate each other and flush up over this pathway from the intestines to the inner ear. As we have seen, stagnant food in infants is ultimately due to their inherently immature and, therefore, weak spleens. Thus, it is no wonder that food stagnation may be aggravated when some children are given solid and, therefore, even more hard-to-digest, food for the first time. This also explains why Chinese children have less problems with ear infections than do Western children. Although there are plenty of things about Chinese culture I do not like, I have to say that their understanding of what is a healthy diet, both for infants and for adults, is way ahead of us in the West.

If this heat condition is treated with antibiotics, the antibiotics do clear the heat, and the condition improves, at least temporarily. The problem is that antibiotics do nothing to help the food stagnation that is typically at the bottom of pediatric earaches and, in fact, contribute to its worsening. This is because antibiotics damage the spleen according to Chinese medical theory. They do this by wiping out all the healthy bacteria that are necessary for the stomach and intestines to function in a healthy, efficient manner. Since the net result of unnecessary or prolonged use of antibiotics is weakening of the spleen, it is easy to see that antibiotics perpetuate a cycle of recurrent inflammation due to food stagnation. Thus each round of antibiotics is followed by another ear infection until finally the parents and their physician don't know what to do besides putting tubes into the eardrums.

Before going any further with this discussion, let me say right here that I am not against all use of antibiotics. Antibiotics have and do save lives. They are a life-saver when they are truly necessary. The problem is that they are given before there is a life-threatening situation. Rather, I believe that antibiotics should be held in reserve as part of a graduating and escalating series of responses. It is my opinion that one should first use safer, more benign, and admittedly less powerful treatments first. Because they are less powerful, they have less potential for unwanted side effects. So first one should use more benign methods like hot and cold compresses (see mumps below for a discussion of how to prepare and administer these) and/or Chinese herbal medicine, both taken orally and applied directly into the ear. For instance, one simple herbal home remedy is to squeeze some fresh peppermint juice and use this juice as eardrops. If these don't get their intended effect and the condition is getting dangerously worse, *then* one can use antibiotics as a last resource.

The good news is that Chinese herbal medicine is very effective for both treating acute earaches as well as preventing recurrent earaches. What's even better, one usually does not need to do an elaborate Chinese medical pattern discrimination, since most infants and toddlers with earaches have the same pattern. The formula that I find most effective are modifications of *Xiao Chai Hu Tang* (Minor Bupleurum Decoction). This formula contains within it herbs to strengthen the spleen, herbs to eliminate dampness and stagnant food from the stomach and intestines, and to clear heat and inflammation. According to Chinese medical theory, these herbal medicinals enter the channels of the stomach and intestines and the gallbladder. These are the channels that encircle and, therefore, treat the ear. This formula has been used in China since at least the second century AD, and statistically it is the most widely prescribed Chinese herbal formula in Japan. Therefore, it has a long history of safe use.

When this formula is used to treat an acute or active current ear infection, ingredients are added to it to help relieve pain and to help clear away inflammation. At the same time, the practitioner may prescribe Chinese herbal eardrops as a local treatment. If there is serious pain, they may even choose to acupuncture the so-called *luo* or connecting vessel of the large intestine. This can help relieve the pain. For the fever, the parent may push down the spinal column from the base of the neck to the sacrum or tailbone, over and over again. And to also help relieve pain, they may massage the forehead and the back of the neck.

Because this condition in children is so intimately connected with their digestive process, it is also absolutely vital that they be fed a clear, bland diet. That means no dairy products like milk or cheese, no greasy, fatty, fried foods, no spicy foods, no sugars and sweets, and no raw, chilled, or frozen foods. This means no raw vegetables and cold drinks on the one hand and frozen yogurt and ice cream on the other. In children with recurrent ear infections, even yeasted wheat products, like bread, should be eliminated.

For the prevention of recurrent ear infections, one can use the basic formula of *Xiao Chai Hu Tang* without a lot of additions or modifications. In this case, the formula should be continued through April of the first year it is begun. The next year, in order to prevent any ear infections, colds, coughs, strep throat, or tonsillitis, this regime is begun again in late September or early October and again continued through April. At the same time, a clear bland diet is essential if the Chinese herbal medicine is to have a chance of achieving its full effect. In Chinese it is said, "Three parts medicine, seven parts nursing." This means that, in the healing of disease, medicine is only responsible for 3/10 of the cure and diet and lifestyle, *i.e.*, nursing, are responsible for 7/10. This is especially true for pediatric ear infections. Without a clear, bland diet as described by Chinese medicine, there is not much chance of a consistent cure.

This also means that the parents are going to have to break the chain of antibiotic use. Commonly this means that the child will have another ear infection soon after the last antibiotics are finished. This is a crucial juncture. If the parents immediately seek remedial treatment with their Chinese medical practitioner, be that a specially modified herbal prescription and eardrops, compresses, infant massage, and/or acupuncture, there is an extremely good chance that antibiotics will not be necessary. In other words, the parents are going to have to bite the bullet and not immediately run for the antibiotics. For some parents who have no previous experience with any other form of health care except modern Western medicine, this may be scary. However, if one immediately goes back to antibiotics, the cycle of repeated ear infections will only continue.

Because this is a potentially frightening position for parents to be in, they should discuss all this thoroughly with their Chinese medical practitioner so that each party knows what treatments will be given in what situations and when it is necessary and appropriate to use antibiotics.

When children are given antibiotics over and over again at a young age, it is my experience as a clinician that this can lead to many years, if not a lifetime, of chronic health problems. In my experience, such children are more prone than others to all sorts of allergies, including hayfever and allergic asthma. They are also more prone to sore throats and tonsillitis. Therefore, I cannot overstress how important it is, in my opinion and experience, not to use antibiotics when not truly necessary.

It is also probably a good idea not to have a nurse or MD look into your child's ears too often. Very often, Western medical practitioners will decide that a child's ears look infected or on the verge of infection and will prescribe antibiotics when the child displays no sign or symptom of an earache other than what is seen through an otoscope (the thing doctors stick in your ear to see your eardrum). This can actually cause problems when there wasn't really a problem to begin with. If a child has constantly bulging eardrums and the doctor says that there is fluid behind the ears and the child shows no other sign or symptom of an infection or inflammation, this can also be treated with Chinese herbal medicine. In this case, your practitioner may choose a formula like *Wu Ling San* (Five [Ingredients] Poria Powder) which seeps away excess fluids and fortifies the spleen, thus undercutting the root mechanisms of ear infections in infants and toddlers.

There are also times when an eardrum does burst. In some cases, the parents may not even have realized that their child was suffering from an earache until after they notice some fluids running from the opening of the ear. Actually, this is the final stage of an ear infection and when this occurs, it marks the resolution of the situation. If this should occur, the Chinese medical practitioner will probably want to prescribe some version of *Huang Qi Jian Zhong Tang* (Astragalus Fortify the Center Decoction). This formula has also been in use from at least the second century AD. It is also appropriate if an eardrum has ruptured and it continues to leak fluids and does not close up as it should. In other words, this formula is designed to promote healing after infection and inflammation are no longer present. It is also important to keep the child's head out of water for 4-6 weeks after an eardrum has ruptured. If water gets in the ear, the child will probably cry from pain and there is the risk of reinfection.

Over the years, I have helped numerous patients and their young charges deal with both acute and chronic ear infections. I know that Chinese herbal medicine combined with a clear, bland diet and avoidance of sugar and antibiotics can prevent and cure ear infections. Feeding a child a clear, bland diet who has been accustomed to sugar and sweets, chilled fruit juices and cold cow's milk, peanut butter and jelly on bread, cheese, and ice cream is no easy task, and I won't kid you by saying that it is. However, I can assure you that it will make a difference in the child's short and long-term health. I really know this works.

Cough (common cold & bronchitis)

When children "catch" the common cold, they usually develop a cough. Cough is one of the most common of all pediatric complaints. Children's coughs often get worse at night. This means that the problem is brought to a head just when the parents are trying to get some much needed sleep. Thus children's coughs are very stressful for the whole family. I have had a lot of clinical experience in treating children's cough, and I feel quite confident in saying that Chinese medicine does a very good job in treating children's cough quickly and effectively, and without side effects.

As with fever above, Chinese medicine divides coughs into two broad types — external and internal. In my experience, however, most infants' coughs are of the internal type. One does not really see the external type until the child is older. This is because the internal patterns mostly have to do with poor spleen function and faulty diet. Therefore, in my practice, what I most often see in infants and toddlers is one of the internal patterns of cough.

There are seven different so-called internal patterns of pediatric cough described in Chinese medicine. These cover cough due to the common cold, cough due to bronchitis, and cough due to asthma. Remember, TCM lays its emphasis on treatment given based on the pattern, not so much on the disease diagnosis. Therefore, it is not so important to the Chinese medical practitioner whether the child has been diagnosed as suffering from bronchitis or asthma.

The first pattern of pediatric cough due to external invasion is called wind cold assailing the lungs. Its symptoms are a mild fever, aversion to draft and chill, absence of perspiration, headache, stuffy nose, clear runny nose, sneezing, cough with thin, white or clear mucus, a thin, white tongue coating, and a floating, tight pulse. The treatment principles for this pattern are to dispel wind and scatter cold, drain the lungs and stop coughing. For children's coughs, I like to use a number of Chinese herbal formulas found in Xiao Shun-qin *et al.*'s *Pediatric Bronchitis: Its TCM Cause, Diagnosis, Treatment & Prevention*. These formulas do not have names, but there is a different formula and various suggested modifications for each pattern discussed. Standard textbook formulas for this pattern include *San Ao Tang* (Three Twisters Decoction) and *Xiao Qing Long Tang* (Minor Blue-green Dragon Decoction). Simple home remedies for this type of cough are to scrape the upper back and shoulders, *i.e.*, *gua sha*, and to give a tea made out of scallions, fresh ginger, and blanched almonds.

The second external invasion pattern, and in my experience with Western children the more common pattern, is wind heat assailing the lungs. Its symptoms are a higher fever and no or only very slight aversion to chill, some sweating but no reduction of the fever when a sweat is broken, headache, yellow, sticky nasal mucus, a red, swollen sore throat, possible swollen tonsils, cough with yellow, sticky phlegm, a red tongue tip with a thin, white or thin, slightly yellow coating, and a floating and rapid pulse. The treatment principles for this pattern are to dispel wind and clear heat, transform phlegm and stop coughing. A standard textbook formula for this type of cough is *Sang Ju Yin* (Morus & Chrysanthemum Drink) with various modifications depending on the presenting signs and symptoms. In this pattern, it is very important not to use a cold bath or cold sponge bath to try to bring down what can be a high fever. What is wanted in this case is for the pores of the skin to be open in order to allow the pathogens to be pushed back out of the body. The application of cold water in this pattern would only shut the pores and drive the pathogens even deeper into the body. *Gua sha* is a good home remedy as is a tea made from peppermint and blanched almonds.

The third pattern of external invasion is wind dryness assailing the lungs. Its symptoms are cough with scanty or no phlegm, a dry, sore throat, a dry mouth and nose, chapped, cracked lips and even an occasional nosebleed, a red tongue with a scanty coating and scanty fluids, and a floating, fine, and rapid pulse. Although the name of this pattern only mentions wind and dryness, in fact, this pattern is a combination of wind, dryness, and heat. The treatment principles for this pattern are to resolve the exterior, clear heat, and moisten dryness. One standard textbook formula for this pattern of cough is *Sang Xing Tang* (Morus & Armeniaca Decoction) with modifications. Because I live and work in high plains/mountain desert conditions, I commonly see and treat this pattern in my patients. However, I do not see it that often in young children because of their tendency to produce so much mucus. When this pattern is seen, use of a humidifier or an old-fashioned steam tent helps to moisten the dryness in the lungs.

The first internal pattern of pediatric cough is phlegm heat accumulation in the lungs. Its symptoms are cough, rough breathing, slimy, white or yellow phlegm, possible fever, possible paroxysmal or spasmodic coughing, a thick, white tongue coating, a red tongue tip and edges, and a slippery, rapid pulse. It is said in Chinese medicine that, "The spleen is the root of phlegm production, while the lungs are the place where phlegm is stored." We have seen above that children have inherently weak spleen's and are, therefore, prone to the development and accumulation of phlegm. Because of the close interrelationship between the spleen and lungs, if the lungs lose their proper function, say, due to a common cold, the spleen may easily become weaker than normal. This is especially so if the child has been eating sugar or sweets or eating chilled dairy products like ice cream or frozen yogurt. Thus this pattern often shows up a few days after the child has attended a birthday party where they ate more sweets and cold dairy products than usual.

The treatment principles for dealing with this type of children's cough are to clear heat and transform phlegm, while also specifically stopping coughing. In the case of phlegm heat accumulation in the lungs, it is very important for the child to be fed a clear, bland diet and to especially avoid sugars and sweets, dairy products, and greasy, fatty, fried foods. Chinese pediatric massage can definitely be of benefit, and some professional practitioners may also do some acupuncture. However, proper diet is the *sine qua non* (can't do without) of this pattern as it is of almost all the cough patterns discussed here. Remember, the spleen is the root of phlegm production, and the lungs are only where it winds up. As soon as we see the word spleen, we know in Chinese medicine that proper diet is going to play a major part in both the condition's prevention and treatment.

The second pattern is heat accumulating in the lungs and stomach. This pattern's symptoms are cough with more yellow, sticky phlegm. The cough may be so bad as to cause vomiting, and if there is vomiting, there is a lot of sticky phlegm mixed in the vomitus. Both sides of the face are red, the hands and feet are hot, and the sick child has a quick temper, cries easily, and sleeps poorly, often kicking off their bed covers. The stools are either dry and hard or are green and loose, in which case, they may occur 2-3 times per day. The urine is yellower than usual and less in amount. The tongue has red edges with a thick, yellow furry coating on top. The pulse is floating and rapid.

This pattern is also due to overeating fried, fatty, greasy foods, sugars and sweets, or simply to overeating. Undigested food stagnates in the stomach and intestines and transforms into evil or pathological heat. This heat moves upward to accumulate in the lungs where it disturbs the lungs proper function. It also disturbs the heart, and this is why there is the irritability and easy crying. Therefore, the treatment principles are to clear heat from the stomach and lungs and to stop coughing. Besides Chinese herbal medicine prescribed professionally for this pattern, Chinese pediatric massage to eliminate food stagnation in the stomach is very useful. Of course, it should go without saying that the diet must be changed to a clear, bland diet without sugars and sweets as well as fried, fatty, greasy foods. Parents should remember that such a list includes chips, french fries, hot dogs and hamburgers, sloppy joe's, etc.

The third pattern is spleen dampness, lung heat. Its signs and symptoms are cough with copious white mucus, heavy breathing, a suffocating feeling in the chest, cloudy runny nose, copious drooling, easy perspiration, poor appetite, a pale face, flaccid muscles and flesh, easily and recurrently getting ill, a tendency to loose stools, when sick, a craving for cold drinks, a pale tongue with a white, wet coating, and a soft, slippery pulse.

These signs and symptoms are due to a combination of heat and phlegm in the lungs but a more pronounced weak spleen. If the child is an infant or very young toddler, they will have the blue vein at the root of their nose between their two eyes. Just as above, this child tends to get ill when their diet is off. The types of things that make them ill are sugar and sweets, diary products, and chilled, cold, frozen drinks and foods — ice cream! These children also tend to get sick when they are fatigued. When they are actually ill, emphasis should be on strengthening the spleen and transforming phlegm, clearing heat and stopping coughing. However, after the cough has abated, diet and pediatric massage designed to strengthen the spleen and improve the digestion is essential.

The fourth pattern is phlegm heat injuring the yin. Yin in this case refers to the healthy moistening fluids of the lungs. If the child has developed phlegm and heat in their lungs and these have not been properly treated and the condition endures for some time, the heat will eventually exhaust and consume the lungs healthy fluids. Thus there will be a combination of symptoms due to the simultaneous presence of heat, phlegm, and dryness. For instance, the child has usually coughed for a long time with little or no phlegm. The cough is more severe in the middle of the night than during the day. The throat is dry, the tongue is red, and there is a lack of coating or fluids on the tongue. The pulse is fine and rapid.

The treatment principles in this case are to enrich yin and clear heat, transform phlegm and stop coughing. Happily, this pattern is not that commonly seen in my experience. Also happily, when it is seen, Chinese medicine treats this pattern where modern Western medicine often fails. If the three preceding patterns are dealt with in an efficient and timely manner, then the cough should not develop into this fourth pattern. One of the times one does see this pattern is after whooping cough or pertussis has gone on for some weeks. A simple Chinese herbal home remedy for this pattern of cough is to make a tea from watercress and blanched almonds. Watercress is cool, clears heat, and moistens the lungs, while almonds transform phlegm, moisten the intestines, and stop coughing. Another simple home remedy is to make a tea from figs, particularly fresh figs if available. Figs clear heat and moisten the lungs and intestines.

The fifth pattern of internal cough is lung qi deficiency. Its signs and symptoms include cough with thin, white or clear, watery phlegm, a weak cough which is worse on exertion or provoked by talking, shortness of breath frequently accompanied by wheezing, low spirits, lack of energy, easy fatigue, spontaneous perspiration or sweating on slight exertion, easy catching cold, a pale face, a pale tongue with a thin, white coating, and a deep, weak pulse. For this pattern, the treatment principles are to supplement and boost the lung qi, transform phlegm and stop coughing. This pattern is seen in children who have been sick a long time. These children should be fed a diet of cooked, warm, nutritious though nevertheless easily digested foods, such as soups, broths, and stews. Spinal pinch-pull up the back can increase basic health and resistance. Because Chinese medicine has a number of herbal medicines which boost and supplement the qi, Chinese herbal medicine is an extremely effective treatment option for this kind of cough, often getting a cure or marked improvement where modern Western medicine has little to offer.

The sixth pattern is lung and kidney deficiency cough. The child coughs and wheezes with copious, thin, white phlegm and much sweating. They feel short of breath, suffocated, and gasp for air, *i.e.*, have asthma. The wings of their nose flare when trying to breathe. Wheezing is provoked by movement and exertion. The child looks listless, they do not like to move about, and they fear cold. Their hands and feet are cold and their urination tends to be frequent, long, and clear. They may also experience incontinence of either urine or stools with a bout of coughing. Their facial complexion is dull, their tongue is pale, and their pulse is deep and fine or deep, slow, and weak. The treatment principles for this type of pediatric cough are to supplement the lungs and to boost the kidneys. This can be done with Chinese herbal medicine. This pattern is often seen in children suffering from chronic bronchial asthma, including allergic asthma. A simple Chinese herbal home remedy for this pattern is to cook mulberries over a low flame down into a syrup with honey added. Then take 2 teaspoons of this syrup 2 times each day. Another possibility is to eat fresh peaches.

The seventh and last internal pattern of pediatric cough is dual deficiency of the lungs and spleen. Its symptoms are cough with thin, white phlegm, shortness of breath, wheezing, frequent catching cold, poor appetite, fatigue, lack of strength, a fat, pale tongue with the marks of the teeth on its edges, a slimy, greasy, white tongue coating, and a deep, relaxed (*i.e.*, almost slow) pulse. This condition is due to constitutional spleen deficiency aggravated by overeating sugars and sweets and cold, chilled foods and drinks. In some ways it is similar to the pattern above in that the patient's symptoms mostly have to do with qi deficiency. However, in this case the two organs which are deficient are the lungs and spleen, while above they are the lungs and kidneys. Therefore, the treatment principles for this pattern are to supplement the lungs and boost the spleen. Because the spleen plays such a pivotal role in the creation of qi in the body, it is vitally important that children with this pattern be fed a diet of cooked, warm, clear, bland but nourishing food. Very young children can also be strengthened by the spinal pinch-pull massage maneuver done daily. Some acupuncturists and professional practitioners of Chinese medicine may also teach parents of children with this pattern how to do moxibustion daily over certain acupuncture points. Moxibustion is the burning of certain Chinese herbs near acupuncture points in order to strengthen the organs and functions connected with those points. In particular, Job's tears barley is believed by Chinese doctors to strengthen both the spleen and the lungs.

As the reader can see, in most of these internal cough patterns, the spleen and, therefore, diet play an important role. "The spleen is the root of phlegm production, while the lungs are where phlegm is stored." This two line verse is the key to diagnosing and treating pediatric cough in my experience. Children's cough can be prevented by feeding them a diet of primarily warm, cooked food which is not too greasy or fatty, not too hot and spicy, and not too much sugar and sweets. In particular, diary products tend to produce phlegm easily because of their very damp, wet nature. While chilled, frozen, and cold foods and drinks easily damage children's fragile spleens and stomachs. So often do children "catch cold" or develop a cough after eating sugars and sweets and soda and ice cream that I routinely ask parents of children with coughs if their child has recently eaten these things. In the United States, I see a huge increase in children's coughs and colds directly after Halloween when children go "trick or treating" for shopping bags of candy and sweets. It is my experience that if parents can control and limit the amounts of sugar and sweets, most pediatric coughs can be prevented.

As an interesting addendum to this discussion of pediatric cough, excessive phlegm can be treated by boiling 57-85g of raw peanuts without their skins briefly in water and then eating the resulting soup. While raw peanuts are believed to help transform and eliminate phlegm, Chinese medicine says that roasted peanuts have the opposite effect — generating more phlegm. Peanut butter is a favorite food of many Western children and peanut butter is made from *roasted* peanuts.

Whooping cough

Whooping cough or pertussis is an acute, infectious, upper respiratory infection due, according to Western medicine, to the *Bordetella pertussis* bacteria. There is also a milder form of this disease caused by *Bordetella parapertussis*. This milder form is called para-pertussis. Children under seven are most susceptible to pertussis and it occurs more often in the late winter and early spring. Although most American children are immu-nized against pertussis, because there is on-going controversy over the safety and effectiveness of the pertussis vaccine, a substantial number of children are not vacci-nated and there are cases of whooping cough in most Western communities. Whooping cough gets its name from the distinctive whooping sound at the end of a series of coughs. There are 5-15 coughs in a row followed by a hurried, deep inhalation or the whoop. These coughs are paroxysmal or spasmodic in nature. Chinese medicine calls whooping cough, *bai ri ke* or hundred day cough. This is because, if left untreated, it tends to persist for three months or 100 days. Whooping cough is a serious disease but it is not necessarily life-threatening. When babies under six months get pertussis, special care must be taken to prevent their inhaling their mucus and vomit and thus asphyxiat-ing themselves. Otherwise, the danger of pertussis is that, *if not properly treated*, it can lead to pneumonia. However, if treated with professionally administered Chinese medicine, that should not happen.

According to Chinese medical theory, whooping cough occurs in children who already have an accumulation of phlegm in their body, and, as we have already seen, such an accumulation of phlegm is due to poor spleen function in turn due to or worsened by faulty diet. If such a child is invaded by an external pathogen, then this external invasion and the accumulation of phlegm already present mutually aggravate each other. Therefore, right away, parents should know that keeping their child's spleen function in healthy shape and keeping phlegm production to a minimum is one way to help prevent your child from developing whooping cough.

Chinese medicine approaches the treatment of pertussis by dividing the course of disease into three stages — the initial stage which typically lasts 10-20 days, the second stage which lasts between 40-60 days, and the recovery stage which lasts between 20-30 days. The pattern associated with the first stage is usually described as cold and phlegm fettering the lungs. Its symptoms are spasmodic cough with thin, watery phlegm, clear, runny nose, a floating, tight pulse, and a white, glossy tongue coating. The treatment principles are to warm the lungs and transform phlegm, normalize the flow of qi and downbear counterflow. Downbear counterflow is a technical term in this case relating to the cough. The lung qi should flow downward, whereas cough is an upward counter-flow of lung qi. Professional practitioners of Chinese medicine typically prescribe some version of *Xiao Qing Long Tang* (Minor Blue-green Dragon Decoction) for this pattern of pertussis.

In the second stage, the main pattern is phlegm heat attaching to the lungs. This implies that phlegm and heat are lingering in the lungs and are reluctant to leave. The symp-toms of this pattern are spasmodic cough with thicker, pastier phlegm which is not easily spit up. Within the phlegm there may be blood. If severe, there is spitting up of blood or a nosebleed. There is also a dry mouth and tongue, thirst with a desire to drink water, a slippery, rapid pulse, and a dry tongue coating. The treatment principles are to clear heat and drain the lungs, stop coughing and transform phlegm. One commonly prescribed formula for this pattern is *Sang Bai Pi Tang* (Morus Bark Decoction) with modifications. A simple Chinese herbal home remedy for this pattern of whooping cough is to boil 15 fresh marigold flower heads in water, mix with a little brown sugar, and drink.

In the third or recovery stage, the main problem is that the disease has gone on for so long, it has damaged the child's righteous or healthy qi. Depending on whether the child tends to run hot or cold and depending upon other factors such as their diet and the height and duration of fever, the two commonly seen patterns during this recovery stage are lung/spleen dual deficiency and yin deficiency. The lung/spleen dual deficiency pattern is characterized by an excessively long recuperation period, a weak cough, scanty, watery phlegm, shortness of breath, a weak voice and disinclination to speak with speaking often provoking a bout of coughing, a pale white facial complexion, diminished appetite, a fine, weak pulse, and a pale tongue with a scanty coating. The treatment principles are to fortify the spleen and harmonize the center, nourish the lungs and stop coughing. A commonly prescribed formula for this pattern of late stage pertussis is *Ren Shen Wu Wei Zi Tang* (Ginseng & Schizandra Decoction) with various modifications as necessary. Children with this pattern obviously need rest and a cooked, warm, nourishing, clear, bland diet. They should not be allowed to eat sugar and sweets or raw, chilled, cold, frozen foods and drinks. Acupuncturists and professional practitioners of Chinese medicine may teach the parents how to do moxibustion at home daily, and a daily administration of spinal pinch pull massage up the spine several times a day can also strengthen the body and its recuperative powers.

The yin deficiency pattern is characterized by a weak, forceless, dry cough, heat in the palms of the hands and soles of the feet, restless sleep and easy waking at night, possible night sweats, irritability, flushed red cheeks, especially in the late afternoon and evening, dry, red lips, a red tongue with a thin, yellow coating, and a rapid, fine, forceless pulse. The treatment principles for this pattern of whooping cough are to enrich yin and moisten the lungs. There are a number of Chinese herbal formulas which may be chosen for these purposes, but a representative one is *Qing Zao Jiu Fei Tang* (Clear Dryness & Rescue the Lungs Decoction) with additions and subtractions depending upon the actual case.

It is interesting to note that Chinese doctors have recently begun adding ingredients to formulas for whooping cough from the antispasmodic category of Chinese medicinals. These are ingredients which are usually used for convulsions, tremors, and paralysis, and are not usually thought of for coughs and lung problems. However, modern Chinese doctors have noticed the spasmodic nature of the cough in whooping cough and have added these antispasmodic ingredients on that basis. These ingredients seem to make formulas for pertussis more effective.

Simple Chinese herbal home remedies for whooping cough are: 1) cooking carrots and red dates (available at Oriental specialty food shops and Chinese apothecaries) into a soup, 2) steaming a lemon with sugar and eating it every morning for whooping cough with excessive phlegm, and 3) taking a 2 teaspoons of a 10-20% garlic solution every two hours. Liquid garlic is available at Western health food stores.

Pediatric pneumonia

Pneumonia in children typically occurs before two years of age and usually in the winter and spring. The general symptoms of pneumonia are fever, a productive cough, shortness of breath, flaring of the wings of the nose when breathing, and cyanotic, *i.e.,* bluish-purplish, lips. Pneumonia, as opposed to bronchitis or bronchial asthma, is diagnosed by the particular crackling, bubbly sounds in the lungs when listened to with a stethoscope and by x-rays showing a cloudy patch on the lungs. In other words, a diagnosis of pneumonia can only be made by a Western MD. There is no traditional Chinese disease category corresponding to pneumonia. Traditionally, it is treated according to the presenting pattern under the heading of cough.

Pneumonia may be caused by direct infection by *Streptococcus pneumoniae* or may be a development from some already existing upper respiratory tract infection which either has not been treated in a timely manner or has not been treated correctly. For instance, pneumonia may result as a complication of measles or whooping cough. Chinese medicine identifies six main patterns of pediatric pneumonia, four of which are excess patterns and two of which are deficiency patterns.

The first pattern is wind cold. Its symptoms are fever with no perspiration, aversion to cold, cough, shortness of breath, no particular thirst, thin, white phlegm, a thin, white or white slimy tongue coating, and a floating, tight pulse. The treatment principles for this pattern are to resolve the exterior with acrid warm medicinals, diffuse the lungs and transform phlegm. A standard formula for this pattern of pediatric pneumonia is *San Ao Tang* (Three Twisters Decoction) with additions and subtractions depending on the case. In addition to Chinese herbal medicine, scraping the upper back (*gua sha*) and acupuncture are useful adjunctive treatments. The patient should be kept under covers in order both to avoid further chill and to promote sweating. Hot, dilute rice soup can also help promote sweating and improve the effect of the herbs. A home remedy for all upper respiratory tract infections characterized as wind cold patterns is to boil several pieces of scallions with some fresh ginger and brown sugar. These ingredients are acrid and warm and thus open or resolve the exterior and warm or scatter cold.

The second pattern is wind heat and, in fact, wind heat is much more commonly seen than wind cold. Its symptoms are fever with sweating or at least slight sweating, thirst, cough with sticky, yellow phlegm, a red tongue with a thin, yellow coating, and a floating, slippery, rapid pulse. The treatment principles for this pattern are to dispel wind and clear heat, diffuse the lungs and transform phlegm. Commonly, *Yin Qiao San* (Lonicera & Forsythia Powder) combined with *Ma Xing Shi Gan Tang* (Ephedra, Armeniaca, Gypsum & Licorice Decoction) with modifications are used to treat this pattern of pediatric pneumonia with Chinese herbal medicine. *Gua sha* of the upper back and shoulders can be used to help resolve the exterior more effectively and rubbing down the center of the spine can help reduce the fever which is higher in this second pattern than the first. For any kind of wind heat pattern of upper respiratory infection (and the reader will come across this pattern a number of times in this section on the diagnosis and treatment of disease), one can make a tea out of fresh peppermint and drink this frequently. In Chinese medicine, peppermint is described as being acrid and cooling. It opens or relieves the exterior and clears heat. Spearmint, on the other hand is acrid and warm and, therefore, should only be used for wind cold patterns as described above.

The third pattern and, in my experience, the most commonly encountered pattern of pediatric pneumonia, is phlegm and heat accumulating in the lungs. We have already discussed this pattern above under cough. The difference in treatment of this pattern when it occurs in pneumonia is simply that more and stronger ingredients may be used as well as ingredients that are known to be specifically effective for the treatment of pneumonia, such as Herba Houttuynia Cordatae (_Yu Xing Cao_).

The fourth pattern of pediatric pneumonia is phlegm dampness stagnating in the lungs. The signs and symptoms of this pattern are cough with copious, white phlegm, shortness of breath, wheezing and dyspnea, the sound of phlegm rattling in the throat, a yellowish face and pale lips, sometimes hot, sometimes cold, a red tongue with a slimy coating, and a slippery pulse. The treatment principles for this pattern are to dry dampness, transform phlegm, and stop cough and wheezing. One standard Chinese herbal approach to the treatment of this pattern is to use a combination of _Xiao Qing Long Tang_ (Minor Blue-green Dragon Decoction) combined with _Er Chen Tang_ (Two Aged [Ingredients] Decoction) with various modifications. This pattern is different from the one above in that there is not so much heat but more phlegm and dampness. As we have already seen, "The spleen is the root of phlegm production, while the lungs are where phlegm is stored." Therefore, in this pattern, a clear, bland diet is especially important as are cooked, warm foods which strengthen the spleen. Dairy products and sugars and sweets as well as raw, cold, chilled, and frozen foods and drinks should be strictly avoided. The yellow face and pale lips are signs in this pattern that the dampness and phlegm are associated with a weak spleen.

If pneumonia is not treated speedily or if the upper respiratory tract infection that has led to pneumonia has endured for some time, pathological heat may have exhausted and consumed the righteous qi of the body. Therefore, the body is too weak to efficiently and effectively fight off the infection. Depending on how high and how prolonged the fever has been and the patients underlying constitutional predisposition, either of two deficiency patterns may present in cases which linger and do not heal.

The first deficiency pattern is yin deficiency with internal heat. We have discussed this pattern above under cough and its treatment principles and treatment plan are essentially the same as discussed above. The second pattern is qi deficiency of the lungs and spleen and we have also discussed this pattern above under cough. In the yin deficiency pattern, a little dairy is actually good, as is a little bit of sweet. More important are nourishing meat broths and eggs. In other words, patients with the yin deficiency pattern need a little more animal protein in order to help recuperate. In the lung/spleen qi deficiency pattern, it is important to avoid sweets and to also avoid raw, cold, chilled, and frozen foods and drinks. In both patterns, adequate rest is absolutely necessary.

For the wind cold, phlegm dampness, and lung and spleen dual deficiency patterns of pneumonia, one can crush and pound together fresh buttercup (Ranunculus) with sugar at a ratio of 10 to 1 respectively. Buttercup is a common perennial garden flower (which should never be taken internally!). This paste is then spread over the area of the chest corresponding to the shadow on the x-ray. This paste should be aged for 1-2 months before use. Otherwise it will tend to cause blisters on the skin. However, since one does not know 1-2 months in advance that they may need this paste, one can still make and use this paste, however knowing in advance that it may cause blistering. As long as such blisters are kept clean and uninfected, this "counterirritation" is actually healing for the pneumonia.

The important thing for parents to know is that Chinese medicine does treat pneumonia without necessarily resorting to antibiotics. As the reader is by now aware, I really do counsel avoiding antibiotics unless truly necessary. Many parents and their MDs, as soon as a diagnosis of pneumonia is made, assume there is no other alternative to antibiotics. Chinese herbal medicine is such an alternative as long as the case is closely monitored by a Western MD. If and when antibiotics become necessary, then they can be used.

Pediatric asthma

Pediatric asthma is mostly an allergic disease. It occurs most frequently in children four or more years of age and occurs more often in the spring and fall. It is characterized by recurrent bouts of an oppressive feeling of tightness in the chest and throat followed by wheezing, shortness of breath, and difficulty breathing. During an attack, the child will not be able to calmly rest while lying down on their back but must often sit up in order to facilitate breathing. Frequently, the asthma spontaneously improves as the child grows older, but may relapse again as an adult if one becomes stressed, run down, has a poor diet, or as one ages. Thus asthma which begins in childhood may often become a life-long problem.

This condition is also characterized by its acute bouts separated by periods of remission, and its TCM treatment takes this into account in terms of pattern discrimination and treatment. During acute attacks, there are two patterns which are distinguished — hot-natured asthma and cold-natured asthma. The symptoms of hot-natured asthma are cough, panting and wheezing, thick, yellow-colored phlegm, fever, a red face, a stuffy, oppressed feeling in the chest, thirst with a desire to drink, reddish yellow urine, dry stools or constipation, a red tongue with a thin, yellow or slimy, yellow coating, and a slippery, rapid pulse. The treatment principles are to clear the lungs, transform phlegm, and stabilize the asthma. This is often treated with the formula, *Ding Chuan Tang* (Calm Asthma Decoction). Since this pattern is one of heat and phlegm, anything which would increase heat in the body, such as hot, spicy foods, or anything which would increase phlegm, such as fatty, greasy foods, sugars and sweets, and dairy products, are contraindicated.

The cold-natured pattern of an acute asthma attack manifests as cough with rapid breathing, the sound of phlegm rattling in the throat, cough with clear, watery, white-colored phlegm, a cold body and no perspiration, a dull, lusterless, "stagnant" facial complexion which may even be a bit bluish green, lack of warmth in the four limbs, no thirst or thirst with a desire for hot drinks only, a thin, white or white, slimy tongue coating, and a floating, slippery pulse. The treatment principles for this pattern are to warm the lungs, transform phlegm, and stabilize asthma. A commonly prescribed and representative formula for this pattern of pediatric asthma is *Xiao Qing Long Tang* (Minor Blue-green Dragon Decoction) with modifications. Obviously, patients with this cold pattern of acute asthma should be kept warm and not be allowed to eat anything cold, frozen, or chilled. Nor should they eat sugar, sweets, or dairy products.

During the remission stage, Chinese doctors try to prevent future asthmatic attacks by building up the body's strength and immunity. Here, we distinguish between three deficiency patterns — lung qi deficiency, spleen qi deficiency weakness, and kidney vacuity not absorbing. The lung qi deficiency pattern is characterized by a dull white or somber white facial complexion, shortness of breath and disinclination to speak, a soft, low voice, fatigue, lack of strength, spontaneous perspiration or sweating on slight movement, fear of chill, lack of warmth in the four limbs, a pale tongue with a thin coating, and a fine, forceless pulse. The treatment principles are to supplement the lungs and secure the defensive. Securing the defensive means to improve the immunity against external pathogens or allergens. A commonly prescribed formula for this pattern is *Yu Ping Feng San* (Jade Wind Screen Powder) with various additions and subtractions.

The spleen qi deficiency weakness pattern mostly manifests as cough with copious phlegm, scanty appetite, a full feeling in the upper abdomen, a yellow, lusterless facial complexion, incomplete stools or loose stools, emaciation, fatigue, lack of strength, a pale tongue with a scanty coating, and a relaxed, *i.e.*, on the verge of slow, forceless pulse. The treatment principles are to fortify the spleen and transform phlegm. Professional practitioners of Chinese medicine commonly prescribe *Liu Jun Zi Tang* (Six Gentlemen Decoction) with modifications for these purposes. Of course, proper diet is vitally important in this pattern and the child should be encouraged to exercise more in order to build up their resistance and strength. Because of their cold nature, many Chinese doctors think that bananas should not be eaten too regularly by persons with a weak spleen and asthma or other lung problems.

In the kidney deficiency not absorbing pattern, the signs and symptoms are a somber or dull white facial complexion, a cold body and fear of chill, lack of warmth particularly in the feet and lower legs, lack of strength in the lower legs, exertion causing heart palpitations and rapid breathing, watery, loose stools, possible bed-wetting at night, a pale tongue with a white coating, and a fine, forceless pulse. The treatment principles are to supplement the kidneys and secure the root. The root has to do with the kidney qi which is rooted in the pelvis or lower abdomen according to Chinese medicine. Probably the most commonly prescribed Chinese herbal formula for this pattern is *Jin Gui Shen Qi Wan* (Kidney Qi Pills [from the book titled *Essentials from the Golden Cabinet*]) with modifications as necessary. Moxibustion over the navel and the lower abdomen is a usual adjunctive treatment and, in children less than six years of age, daily spinal pinch pull massage can help strengthen the constitution.

As one can see, the emphasis with asthma should be on prevention. Because this is an allergic condition, diet is vitally important. For more information on diet and allergies see the section on allergies below. It is also true that emotional stress plays its part in most cases of asthma as does a history of antibiotic use leading to chronic candidiasis. So many of my son's friends can't come to our house because they have allergic asthma triggered by animal hair and dander. These are the same children whose parents do not seem to care how much sugar, ice cream, and soda they consume and who run to the MD for antibiotics at the first sign of an ear infection or sore throat. Having suffered from pediatric asthma and allergies myself as a child, I know what a drag this is, and I also know that much of this suffering is entirely unnecessary if one pays attention to proper diet and avoids antibiotics if at all possible.

Swollen glands (strep throat & tonsillitis)

In the back of the throat and under the jaws there are a number of salivary and lymph glands. These may become infected and/or enlarged. In some cases, if the child is taken to a Western MD or clinic and a throat culture is done, the Western medical diagnosis is a strep (short for streptococcus) infection. Unless the parent refuses, children who test positive for strep are given antibiotics. In my generation, children with recurrent sore throats and swollen glands or tonsillitis eventually had their tonsils removed. Happily today, Western MDs don't seem to be so quick to recommend a tonsillectomy. In most cases of sore throat, swollen glands, and tonsillitis, antibiotics and surgery are not necessary and these conditions can be treated successfully by Chinese medicine, including Chinese herbal medicine and acupuncture.

Most sore throats, at least in their first day or so, tend to be identified as a wind heat external invasion in TCM. There is a fever, no or slight chills, slight perspiration, stuffy and/or runny nose, possible cough, a thin, white or just barely yellow tongue coating, and a floating, rapid pulse. The treatment principles for this pattern are to resolve the exterior, dispel wind, and clear heat. If the sore throat is more serious, then the Chinese practitioner may also say that there are heat toxins. In that case, then the principle of resolving toxins is added to the above list. In this case, there are a number of formulas which may be prescribed which effectively treat this beginning stage of an upper respiratory tract infection affecting the throat and glands. For instance, if there is fever and sore throat but no cough, the practitioner may prescribe *Yin Qiao Jie Du Tang* (Lonicerae & Forsythia Resolve Toxins Decoction), while if there is a cough, they may prescribe *Sang Ju Yin* (Morus & Chrysanthemum Drink).

If swollen glands are more obvious and/or the tonsils are visibly inflamed with white, purulent patches, the Chinese medical practitioner will emphasize heat or fire toxins even more. In this case, they may recommend *Liu Shen Wan* (Six Spirits Pills). This formula is very effective for treating sore throat, including tonsillitis. Acupuncturists will probably recommend bleeding two points on the sides of the thumbnails. I have seen many cases of acute tonsillitis and severe sore throat while an intern in China treated by letting a drop of blood from these two points and the patient reporting relief from their sore throat almost immediately thereafter. If there is fever, this can be treated by massaging repeatedly down the center of the spine. In addition, alternating hot and cold compresses around the throat (15 minutes hot, 5 minutes cold) can provide symptomatic relief and hasten recovery.

If the fever goes down and the glands are no longer hot and painful but are still swollen and hard, this is diagnosed as phlegm nodulation. In this case, the Chinese medical practitioner will probably write a prescription containing Chinese herbs to soften the hard, transform phlegm, and scatter nodulation. In this case, it is important for the child not to eat any dairy products, any fried or fatty foods, or any sugar and sweets, all of which can aggravate phlegm conditions according to Chinese medical theory.

For children with a history of recurrent tonsillitis who have been treated repeatedly with antibiotics and are facing an imminent tonsillectomy, a radical change to a clear, bland diet and the use of a preventive formula such as *Xiao Chai Hu Tang* (Minor Bupleurum Decoction, discussed above under ear infections) can break this cycle and save the tonsils. Usually I recommend the child taking such a formula until April of the current year and then starting again in late September and again taking it until April. It is my assumption that the body has evolved the tonsils for a good reason and that removing them unless absolutely necessary is not a good idea for the long-term health and immunity of the person.

Strep throat

When throat cultures are done and they come back positive for strep, then the parents face a dilemma. The Western clinician will say that antibiotics are absolutely necessary in order to avoid scarlatina or what used to be called scarlet fever. It is true that some strep infections, left untreated, may develop into scarlatina and that scarlatina, if left untreated or is poorly treated, may develop into rheumatic fever affecting the heart. No one, least of all myself, wants to see any child develop rheumatic heart disease which can weaken the heart for the rest of one's life. However, neither do I want to see children receive antibiotics unless absolutely necessary, since I have seen too many long-term negative repercussions from these, such as enduring food, respiratory, and skin allergies and eventual autoimmune conditions. So what is a parent to do?

The key is the word untreated. If a strep infection is left untreated, then yes, it may potentially, although by no means always, develop into scarlatina and even eventually into rheumatic fever affecting the heart. But there is more than one way to treat a strep infection of the throat. Antibiotics are one way. They effectively knock out the strep, but they also knock out all the good bacteria and lead to an imbalance in the bacteria and fungi in the gut which then may lead to chronic allergies which may lead to autoimmune disorders. Chinese herbal medicine is another way of treating strep infections — but a way without the negative side effects of antibiotics. A number of the Chinese medicinals which are used for treating throat infections, swollen glands, and tonsillitis have been proven to have broad spectrum antibiotic ability, in some cases even surpassing antibiotics in efficiency. In particular, a number of Chinese medicinals for these problems have been shown in laboratory tests that they do kill the streptococcus bacteria, such as Radix Isatidis Seu Baphicacanthi (*Ban Lan Gen*), Rhizoma Coptidis Chinensis (*Huang Lian*), Radix Scutellariae Baicalensis (*Huang Qin*), Herba Houttuynia Cordatae (*Yu Xing Cao*), Fructuficatio Lasioshaerae (*Ma Bo*), Herba Cum Radice Taraxaci Mongolici (*Pu Gong Ying*), Fructus Forsythiae Suspensae (*Lian Qiao*), and Flos Lonicerae Japonicae (*Yin Hua*). In other words, Chinese herbal medicines can definitely treat strep infections without antibiotics. And since these Chinese medicinals are always administered as part of a balanced formula, they do not damage the spleen the way antibiotics do.

In like manner, Chinese medicine also treats scarlatina. In other words, even if a strep infection did progress to scarlet fever, it does not necessarily have to wind up damaging the heart. The issue is whether or not there is an effective treatment preventing the disease from going deeper into the body. If treatment effectively cures the disease without either short or long-term side effects, then that is the best, and that can be accomplished with Chinese herbal medicine for these problems. On the other hand, if for some reason, the Chinese herbal medicine does not get an entirely satisfactory effect and the child's condition is getting worse, one can always fall back on antibiotics at that point, after one has given safer, less harmful treatments first. Thus the issue is not simply whether to give antibiotics, but when to give antibiotics.

In order to allay parents' fears about strep throat, I would like to quote Robert S. Mendelsohn, MD, from his excellent book, *How to Raise a Healthy Child...In Spite of Your Doctor*:

> First, you should be aware that sore throats, most of the time, are caused by viruses for which Modern Medicine has no cure...
>
> Secondly, you should know that taking a culture to determine the presence of "strep" is a waste of your money and the doctor's time. It will *not* prove beyond doubt that your child has, or does not have, a strep infection...
>
> Third, the chances that your child will experience rheumatic fever, even if he has a strep infection, are extremely remote. During a quarter of a century in a pediatric practice that had more than 10,000 patient contacts a year, I saw only one case of rheumatic fever. In real life, the threat of rheumatic fever does not exist in most populations. The disease is rarely seen except among malnourished children living in the crowded conditions associated with desperate poverty.

Lack of appetite

Sometimes children lose their appetite for relatively long periods of time and may even refuse to eat. This mostly occurs in children from 1-6 years of age. Although the child eats very little, they are, nevertheless, energetic and seem in good spirits. If lack of appetite and refusal to eat continues for a long time, it may affect the child's growth and development. There are three basic patterns which Chinese pediatric texts associate with pediatric anorexia or lack of appetite in children.

The first pattern is called loss of fortification in spleen transportation. This can also be called food stagnation loss of appetite. It is due to the child being overfed. Because of an inherently weak spleen, the spleen cannot digest all this food and thus it stagnates within the stomach and intestines. The symptoms of this pattern are a lusterless facial complexion, no thought for food or drink, no taste in eating or drinking, refusal to eat or drink, a somewhat emaciated body, a distended abdomen, flatulence, possible bad breath, basically normal urination and defecation, a thin, white, slimy tongue coating, and a slippery, forceful pulse. The treatment principles for this pattern of lack of appetite are to harmonize the spleen and strengthen transportation.

A commonly prescribed Chinese herbal formula for the treatment of this pattern of lack of appetite is *Qu Mai Zhi Zhu Wan* (Massa Medica, Hordeus, Aurantium & Atractylodes Pills) with modifications. Massaging the abdomen with small clockwise circles within the large circles can help transport and conduct the food through the intestines. However, it is important not to force the child to eat if they do not want to. After all, this condition is due to the child's overeating. It is also possible for an acupuncturist or professional practitioner of Chinese medicine to do acupuncture at the so-called *Si Feng* or Four Winds points. These are points in the middle of the creases of the knuckles of the four fingers on the palm side of each hand. Needling each of these can help move stagnation and improve the appetite.

The second pattern is spleen and stomach qi deficiency. In this case, the spleen and stomach simply are too weak to digest food and drinks. The difference between this and the preceding pattern is that in this case there are no particularly pronounced symptoms of food stagnation. Rather the signs and symptoms have to do with fatigue and lack of warmth. For instance, there is a somewhat depressed spirit, a sallow yellow facial complexion, lack of appetite, refusal to eat, when the child eats, there tends to be loose stools soon afterwards with undigested food in the stools, easy perspiration, a pale tongue with a thin, white coating, and a forceless pulse. If the child is still an infant or young toddler, there will likely be a visible blue vein at the root of the nose. The treatment principles for this pattern are to fortify or strengthen the spleen and boost the qi. One commonly used formula for this condition is *Shen Ling Bai Zhu San* (Ginseng, Poria & Atractylodes Powder) with modifications to fit the individual case. Moxibustion over the navel can be a useful adjunctive treatment, and when the child eats, they should not be allowed to eat raw, chilled, cold, or frozen foods or drinks on the one hand or sugars and sweets on the other. A simple Chinese herbal home remedy for this pattern of pediatric lack of appetite is to drink a tea made from 20 cloves and some black (Chinese call it red) tea.

The third pattern of childhood lack of appetite is called stomach yin insufficiency. This pattern typically manifests after a febrile disease, such as measles. In this case, the heat of the fever has consumed and dried up the healthy fluids of the stomach. If these fluids within the stomach are insufficient, the stomach cannot perform its function of receiving and taking in foods. The symptoms of this pattern are a dry mouth and a tendency to drink a lot yet no desire to eat food, dry skin, dry stools, a mirror-like or shiny tongue with a peeled coating or a bright red tongue with a scanty coating and scanty fluids, and a fine pulse. The treatment principles for this pattern are to nourish the stomach and foster yin. Professional practitioners of Chinese medicine accomplish this by prescribing Chinese herbal formulas such as *Yang Wei Zeng Jin Tang* (Nourish the Stomach & Increase Fluids Decoction).

Constipation

It is interesting to note that not a single one of the dozen or so Chinese pediatric texts I have in my clinical library lists constipation as a pediatric condition. In general it is true that infants tend to suffer more from diarrhea than from constipation. However, constipation may occur in children either as a major complaint or as part of some other disease. Because the free and regular flow of the bowels is an important component of good health, some mention of constipation is appropriate even though this topic does not appear in Chinese pediatric texts.

Sometimes newborn infants who are breast-fed can go for days without having a bowel movement. I have discussed this condition with both MDs and midwives and everyone I have talked to has said that, if the baby is being breast-fed, and there are no other signs or symptoms that anything is wrong, then there is nothing to worry about even if the baby goes for five, six, or seven days without a bowel movement. However, Chinese doctors often recognize signs and symptoms of imbalance that Western clinicians overlook.

Therefore, if you have a newborn child who has gone several days without a bowel movement, there are two things you can check. First, is there any bad breath? A baby's breath should smell sweet. If the breath smells bad, then this is a main symptom of food stagnation. Such a food stagnation pattern would be corroborated by a purplish, larger than normal vein at the base of the index finger and possible lack of appetite with vomiting of curdled milk. If there is constipation due to food stagnation, then one can rub the abdomen with clockwise small circles within the large circles. This promotes the movement of food through the intestines. Professional practitioners may also recommend using a Chinese herbal formula such as *Bao He Wan* (Protecting Harmony Pills) with various modifications to promote the movement of food through the intestines and to eliminate stagnation. A warm water enema is also a possibility.

If, on the other hand, the child has a visible blue vein at the root of their nose, tends to have cold hands and feet, and seems lethargic, this suggests the pattern of spleen deficiency. In this case, there are lack of bowel movements because the spleen is too weak to promote the transportation and conveyance of the food through the digestive tract. In this case, the treatment principles are to strengthen the spleen and supplement the qi. This can be done either by rubbing the abdomen with counterclockwise small circles within the larger circle, by giving Chinese herbal formulas such as *Xiang Sha Liu Jun Zi Tang* (Auklandia & Amomum Six Gentlemen Decoction) with modifications, or by doing moxa over the navel.

When older children become constipated, this is usually due to heat in the stomach and intestines which causes "binding" of the intestines. In this case, there may be bad breath, a reddish tongue with a thick, dryish, yellow coating, a reddish face, possible abdominal cramps, possible canker sores, and a rapid, slippery, wiry pulse. In this case, constipation can be the major complaint in and of itself, or it may be an accompanying symptom of some other disease, such as a cold with fever, a bad sore throat, and swollen glands. The treatment principles for this type of constipation are to clear heat and drain the bowels.

118

One can do this by giving an enema and/or one can administer a Chinese herbal formula such as *Ma Zi Ren Wan* (Cannabis Seed Pills) or *Xiao Cheng Qi Tang* (Minor Support the Qi Decoction) with various modifications.

If the child is under six years of age, rubbing the abdomen with small clockwise circles within the large circles can also help drain the bowels. A simple Chinese herbal home remedy for heat constipation is to cut up 100g of white Oriental radish, usually sold under its Japanese name, *daikon*, and squeeze out the juice. Then mix with some honey and administer daily. Another simple herbal home remedy is to drink 1 glass of grapefruit juice every morning at breakfast. Grapefruit juice is considered cold in nature.

In elementary school-aged children, insuring that the bowels are not "knotted and bound" due to heat in the stomach and intestines is one way of insuring the child does not get sick with some febrile or feverish disease. This is the truth behind some parents traditionally giving a child an enema at the first sign of getting ill. However, this is really only a good thing to do if the child shows symptoms of excess heat rather than spleen deficiency.

Cold sores

Some children are plagued with cold sores which occur periodically on or around their mouths. These sores are red, inflamed, and blistery. Eventually, crusts and scabs are formed. According to Western medicine, these are due to infection by the *Herpes simplex* virus which becomes active when the person has a cold or flu. However, they may occur even when the child appears otherwise healthy. In Chinese medicine, such cold sores are called *re qi chuang* or hot qi sores. This underscores that their occurrence has something to do with an accumulation of evil or pathological heat in the body. In children, this heat is usually located in the stomach and intestines. This heat is due to overeating in general and to overeating greasy, fatty, fried, or hot, spicy foods in particular. This heat then floats upward to accumulate in the lungs. Commonly there is a reddish tongue with a yellow coating and a rapid, slippery pulse.

According to TCM, the usual treatment principles for this condition are to clear heat and dispel wind. One commonly prescribed Chinese herbal formula which treats this condition is *Xin Yi Qing Fei Yin* (Magnolia Flower Clear the Lungs Drink) with modifications. If there is constipation, an enema can also be helpful for draining heat from the stomach and intestines by promoting bowel movements.

Bed-wetting

Bed-wetting refers to the involuntary discharge of urine during sleep at night in children over 3 years of age. It is mainly due to the inherent immaturity of the kidneys in children. The kidneys control growth and development according to Chinese medicine. For instance, one's permanent teeth and puberty are both signs of the maturation of the Chinese concept of the kidneys. As in Western medicine, the kidneys are also responsible for urination. However, pediatric enuresis, as this condition is technically called, may also be due to spleen and lung deficiency or damp heat. Therefore, the professional practitioner needs to be able to distinguish these three different patterns and give different treatment for each one.

For instance, the signs and symptoms of kidney deficiency bed-wetting include nighttime enuresis 1-2 or more times each night, frequent, clear urination, a pale facial complexion, a tendency to low back or knee soreness or weakness, possible chilled limbs and a fear of cold, and a pale tongue with a thin, white coating. Symptoms of spleen and lung qi deficiency include episodic bed-wetting after or secondary to some other disease, frequent but scanty urination, a pale complexion, fatigue, lassitude of the spirit (meaning a dispirited face or affect), easy sweating on slight or even no exertion, loose stools, and a pale tongue with a thin, white coating. While the symptoms of damp heat pattern bed-wetting are small amounts of dark-colored, strong-smelling urine, irritability, talking in one's sleep, grinding of teeth while asleep, and red lips and tongue.

In each of these three cases, a different treatment is necessary. If treated by Chinese herbal medicine, the kidney deficiency type is treated by formulas such as *Jin Suo Gu*

Jing Wan (Golden Lock Secure the Essence Pills). The spleen and lung deficiency pattern is treated by modifications of *Bu Zhong Yi Qi Tang* (Supplement the Center & Boost the Qi Decoction). A simple Chinese herbal home remedy for this pattern of bed-wetting is to make a tea out of cinnamon and licorice and add 2 teaspoons of molasses. And the damp heat pattern is treated by modifications of formulas such as *Long Dan Xie Gan Tang* (Gentiana Drain the Liver Decoction). In clinical practice, it is most common to see cases of enuresis due to kidney deficiency, and, quite frankly, such cases may only present with a scant few of the symptoms listed. Happily, when due to this mechanism, *Jin Suo Gu Jing Wan*, which comes as little round pills which are easy for young children to swallow, usually provides cheap, easy, and effective treatment.

It is also possible to treat the kidney deficiency pattern of enuresis with daily Chinese infant massage. In this case, one does the spinal pinch pull maneuver 3-5 times and then massages the lower abdomen. Some practitioners treat enuresis with acupuncture and this is often effective, although, for obvious reasons, it is not my first choice. In both the kidney deficiency and the spleen/lung deficiency patterns, it is important for the child to be fed a cooked, clear, bland diet. In the case of kidney vacuity, they should especially stay away from chilled drinks and frozen foods. In the spleen lung deficiency type, the child should be kept away from sugars and sweets. While in the damp heat type, the child should be kept from greasy, fatty, fried, and hot, spicy foods. Children with the damp heat pattern are also typically angry over something, and this should be taken into account in their treatment.

Some parents both in China and the West try to shame their children into stopping their bed-wetting, but this is seldom the answer. If the child has weak kidneys, the fear of the parents anger or disdain will only further damage the kidneys according to Chinese medicine. While children with damp heat enuresis in part due to anger and frustration will obviously only get worse in response to their parents' anger and frustration.

Obviously, if a child is having trouble with bed-wetting, they should not be allowed to drink too much in the evening, and the parents should make sure the child empties their bladder before bed each evening. In addition, if due to kidney deficiency or

121

lung/spleen deficiency, the child should not be allowed to become too fatigued before going to bed. Overfatigue only results in further weakening of the kidneys, spleen, and lungs.

Impetigo

Impetigo is a contagious, blistery, skin disease which is mostly seen in children. From the Western medical point of view, it is due to a bacterial infection. It is characterized by clusters of red water blisters mostly occurring on the arms, legs, and face. When the blisters break, they ooze a thin, honey-colored fluid which, when it dries, forms crusts around the lesions. Because of this yellow-colored exudate, impetigo is traditionally called "yellow fluid sores" or "pus-dripping sores" in Chinese. This disease mostly occurs in the summertime.

In Chinese medicine, this disease is mainly due to damp heat attacking and accumulating in the skin. Therefore, it typically occurs during seasons or in locales where there is a preponderance of dampness and heat, such as the summer. Although this disease is seen as an invasion of external dampness and heat, children with a propensity to be damp and hot internally are more susceptible to this condition, and dampness and heat accumulate internally in children primarily due to their weak spleens and faulty diet. Therefore, in order to prevent your child from contracting impetigo, it is important to foster a healthy spleen and to promote a clear, bland diet. One can fortify the spleen by doing daily infant massage as described above. A clear, bland diet of primarily cooked foods, low in fats and greases and low in sugars and sweets, both fortifies the spleen *and* helps to prevent the accumulation of dampness and heat internally.

If your child does "catch" impetigo, it is important that the lesions be lightly covered with a gauze bandage, since the lesions will spread wherever the yellowish fluids touch. This means that other children should not come in physical contact with either the lesions themselves or the suppurative fluid. It also means that the child must be kept from scratching these lesions. If the lesions are touched, one should immediately wash.

Since impetigo often occurs secondary to scratching a small cut or insect bite with dirty hands, children should be taught to wash their hands frequently and also not to scratch small cuts and bites, since this may lead to infection.

Chinese medicine treats this condition through the internal administration of various herbal decoctions. For instance, your practitioner may choose to use versions of either *Qing Pi Chu Shi Yin* (Clear the Spleen & Eliminate Dampness Drink) or *Er Miao San* (Two Wonders Powder). The practitioner will vary these prescriptions depending upon the exact location of the lesions, their physical appearance, and other factors, such as itching. In addition, your practitioner will also probably prescribe a Chinese herbal wash or lotion. If the lesions are weeping and flowing, it is important not to use an oil-based ointment. This can trap the dampness and heat in the skin and actually cause the lesions to spread and worsen.

In terms of Chinese dietary therapy, a dilute soup or porridge made out of mung beans is useful to help clear damp heat from the child's system. This can be given preventively during hot damp summer weather or remedially if your child develops this condition. Another possibility is to feed your child a dilute porridge made out of Job's tears barley. This is also called Coix by Western practitioners and is available at both health food and Oriental specialty food stores.

If this condition becomes chronic, the scaly, sticky lesions may cover large areas which then do not easily heal. Accompanying symptoms include thirst but no particular desire to drink, fatigue, possible shortness of breath, restlessness, disturbed sleep, a light red tongue with thin or scanty coating, and a fine pulse. These signs and symptoms are due to prolonged dampness and heat damaging the qi and yin of the body. Thus there is a combination of lingering damp heat mixed with yin and qi deficiency. Although this may sound bad, the good news is that this is exactly the kind of condition that Chinese medicine excels at treating. When this pattern appears, your child's practitioner will want to prescribe a combination of Chinese herbs which supplement the qi and fortify the spleen at the same time as enriching yin and clearing and eliminating dampness and heat. For instance, they may choose to prescribe some version of *Shen Qi Zhi Mu Tang* (Codonopsis, Astragalus & Anemarrhena Decoction).

Allergies

In my experience, allergies in children are due to two main causes. The first cause is dietary. Either solid foods were not introduced properly or the child has been allowed to eat the wrong diet. As discussed above, solid foods should only be introduced when the child is old enough to grab for them off their parents' plates. This typically corresponds to the first teething around five months or so. When introducing foods, it is important to only introduce one food at a time. That way, if there is a negative reaction due to the child's digestion not being ready to handle that food, it can be identified and withdrawn until the digestion has matured. If the food is continued to be fed to the child and they really are not digesting it, then the child will tend to become reactive to that food.

In addition, if the child is fed a diet high in sugars and sweets, this will weaken their spleen and cause an accumulation of dampness within the body. If this dampness lingers and accumulates, it will typically give rise to damp heat in the intestines. This damp and hot environment then provides the perfect breeding ground for overgrowths of yeast and fungi. These move outside the intestines. As they do so, they cause the intestinal lining to become more permeable, and so large food molecules which should not enter the blood stream do, where they provoke immune or allergic responses. Also, when these yeasts and fungi move outside the gut and into the body, they eventually die. When they die their proteins are also recognized as foreign and provoke immune or allergic responses.

The other main mechanism for causing allergic states in the body is antibiotics which also, in their own way, foster overgrowths of yeast and fungi. Whether due to faulty diet or to antibiotics, overgrowths of yeast and fungi are directly responsible for the body's becoming allergic or hypersensitive to things it should not ordinarily be allergic to. These may be food allergies, or airborne, upper respiratory allergies, such as hayfever or allergic asthma, or they could be types of allergic dermatitis, such as hives, eczema, and psoriasis.

All of these diseases can be treated according to their pattern discrimination with professionally prescribed Chinese herbal medicine. Since these conditions tend to be complicated, there is little that I can tell parents in terms of home care or self-treatment. However, since diet is such an important part of such allergic conditions, if the parents adopt a clear, bland diet for the child, this will go a long way to solving any of these problems. And, in my experience, none of these problems can be lastingly cured with acupuncture and/or Chinese herbal medicine alone if the diet is not taken care of.

What is the clear, bland diet in terms of allergic diseases? I believe this is so important that I cannot overstate or explain this concept too often. It means eating cooked foods at a warm temperature. Remember, for the spleen to do its work with maximum efficiency, all food in the stomach must be turned into 100° soup. It means eating a diet high in grains and complex carbohydrates. But these grains must be well cooked and/or milled in order for them to be easily digestible. The main grain should be rice since it is so hypoallergenic. It means a diet high in beans and some nuts and seeds. It means a diet high in vegetables and fruits, but preferably cooked for infants and toddlers. It means a little bit of animal protein from time to time.

What should be minimized are sugars and sweets *from all sources.* In my experience, sugar from fruit juice or honey is just as bad as white or refined sugar. A glass of fruit juice has as much or more sugar than a candy bar. Only minimal dairy products, like milk and yogurt, should be eaten. When dairy products are eaten, they should be eaten warm or at least room temperature. The diet should be low in fats and oils and low or even free from foods made through fermentation or which are easily contaminated by yeasts and molds. This means that the child should not eat anything made with yeast, such as bread and cheese, anything with vinegar, or any food which gets moldy easily. Apples don't mold easily but peaches, strawberries, and most melons do, and the hazy outer layer of a grape skin is mold.

Such a clear, bland, hypoallergenic diet is a big change for many children and adults alike. But it is the key to curing so many chronic, otherwise knotty and difficult to treat diseases. When one switches to a diet like this, there may be an initial aggravation as many of the yeasts and fungi in the body die off due to lack of nutrients (read sugar). However, by the end of the first week, there should be obvious improvement.

However, although there can be startling improvement in only a few weeks, this diet must be preserved if it is going to have lasting effect. If it is not adhered to for at least 3 months, its effects will only be very short-lived. If one can keep it up for 6 months, there will be a much better foundation with less tendency to slip backwards. In actual fact, although one can eventually eat aggravating foods from time to time, this is the diet that is healthiest for the majority of people living in temperate climates. This diet has recently been promoted by the U.S. Department of Agriculture with their food pyramid. It is also very similar to the Pritikin diet, the Macrobiotic diet, and the Mediterranean diet at least in its broad outlines.

A simple home treatment for all kinds of allergies is to do cupping over the navel. Cupping is one of the adjunctive external treatments of acupuncture and Chinese medicine. It consists of using a small glass jar, such as an empty jam jar, and a flame in order to make a vacuum with the jar. This vacuum pulls up the skin underneath the opening of the jar so that the jar sticks firmly to the skin. This treatment should be learned from an acupuncturist or other professional practitioner of Chinese medicine. Although it is not difficult to do, one really does need to see it done in order not to burn the child's skin. When cupping such as this is done over the navel, the cup is left in place for 5 minutes and then removed. This is repeated for 3-5 times per session and one session is done per day for several days. This treatment is not appropriate for infants, but can be quite good for young children with all sorts of allergies.

So if your child suffers from upper respiratory, food, or skin allergies or from any autoimmune disease, my advice is to see a well-trained professional practitioner of Chinese medicine *and* to adopt a clear, bland, spleen-strengthening, dampness and phlegm-eliminating, yeast-free, hypoallergenic diet.

Pediatric eczema

Eczema refers to a superficial inflammation of the skin characterized by redness, swelling, blisters, oozing, crusting, scaling, and usually itching. Pediatric eczema is divided into two main patterns in Chinese medicine. There is a damp heat brewing and steaming pattern and a spleen deficiency/blood deficiency pattern. The damp heat brewing and steaming pattern describes eczematous lesions which begin as a red rash. Over time, this rash develops blisters which eventually burst and weep. If these are scratched, a secondary infection may easily occur. The treatment for this first kind of pediatric eczema are to clear heat, disinhibit dampness, and dispel wind. One commonly used Chinese herbal formula for this pattern of pediatric eczema is *Bi Xie Shen Shi Tang* (Dioscorea Hypoglauca Seep Dampness Decoction) with modifications. Patients with this type of eczema must avoid sugar and sweets, anything made through fermentation, and anything that molds easily, while they should eat a cooked, warm, clear, bland, anti-candidal, hypoallergenic diet. Simple Chinese herbal home remedies for this pattern of eczema are a tea made out of Job's tears barley and mung beans; a tea made out of dandelion and corn silks; or a tea made out of aduki beans, Job's tears barley, and cornsilk. Externally, one can wash the affected area with equal portions of salt and borax dissolved in warm water and applied 2-3 times per day.

The second type or pattern of pediatric eczema is spleen deficiency/blood deficiency. This is characterized by a red, swollen rash which is scaly and hard. Itching is relatively mild. There may be a yellow-colored, fatty exudate. This pattern of eczema is actually the subacute or chronic form, while the damp heat pattern describes the acute or active phase. The treatment principles are to fortify the spleen and dry dampness, nourish the blood and dispel wind. *Ping Wei San* (Level [or Calm] the Stomach Powder) combined with *Si Wu Tang* (Four Materials Decoction) with modifications would be a representative formula for this pattern.

In both these patterns, the spleen plays the pivotal role. The presence of damp heat smoldering in the skin is due to poor spleen function. In Chinese medicine, the spleen is responsible for transforming and transporting body fluids. Damp heat occurs in infants and children because of weak spleen function compounded by faulty diet. Dampness accumulates and obstructs the free flow of warm qi which then backs up and turns into heat. This heat commingles with this dampness and thus there is damp heat. In the second pattern, spleen deficiency and weakness give rise to blood deficiency. In Chinese medicine, blood is made out of the essence of food and liquids digested and refined by the spleen. Because the blood nourishes and irrigates the skin, if there is blood deficiency, the skin may become dry, scaly, and itchy.

Therefore, in both patterns, a spleen-strengthening, dampness-eliminating diet is essential. This is the clear, bland diet described above with emphasis on avoiding sugars and sweets, fermented foods, and foods which mold easily. This then is an anti-candidal, hypoallergenic diet as well. Locally, there are Chinese herbal formulas for external application to the eczematous lesions to help them heal more quickly. Your Chinese medical practitioner can select one for your child's appropriate pattern. It is important in the damp heat brewing and steaming stage not to use an oil-based external application, whereas in the dry, scaly stage where there is either little or no weeping, an oil-based formula in order to moisten dryness is just what is needed. A simple Chinese herbal home remedy for wet, weeping eczema is to grate a raw potato and apply as a poultice to the affected area held in place by cotton gauze. This poultice is then changed every three hours.

Pediatric hives

Hives or urticaria are raised weals on the skin. They can be large or small, red or white, all over the body or only in a very localized area. They develop quickly and can also disappear quickly. Most often they are a type of allergic response. Children are especially susceptible to hives because their skin is believed to be looser and less densely packed than adults'. Therefore, they are more easily invaded by evil winds. However, evil wind is only a poetic way of referring to an unseen pathogen. In Chinese pediatrics, there are three main patterns describing hives in children.

The first pattern is wind cold. Its symptoms are pale-colored weals which get worse on exposure to chill or wind. They also tend to be worse in the winter and better in the summer. The tongue has a thin, white, possibly slimy coating, while the pulse is soggy and relaxed (*i.e.*, on the verge of slow). The treatment principles for this pattern of pediatric hives are to dispel wind and scatter cold, and regulate and harmonize the constructive and defensive. The constructive and defensive are two different layers of the qi. What this means is that the defensive layer is not keeping out potential pathogens the way it should. Therefore, the defensive layer of the qi is too permeable. Professional practitioners of Chinese herbal medicine commonly prescribe *Gui Zhi Tang* (Cinnamon Twig Decoction) with modifications for this type of hives. Children with this type of hives should not be allowed to eat or drink anything chilled, frozen, or cold.

The second pattern is wind heat. Its symptoms are red-colored weals which feel burning hot and which itch extraordinarily. They are worse on exposure to heat and are worse in the summer and better in the winter. The tongue has a thin, yellow coating, and the pulse is floating and rapid. The treatment principles are to dispel wind and clear heat, disinhibit dampness and stop itching. *Xiao Feng San* (Dispersing Wind Powder) with additions and subtractions is a commonly prescribed Chinese herbal formula for this pattern of pediatric hives. Children with this pattern should not be allowed to eat anything hot or spicy, nor should they eat chicken, shrimp, shellfish in general, strawberries, chocolate, and other foods which Chinese medicine regards as likely to cause hot-natured allergic reactions.

The third pattern is intestine and stomach damp heat. Its symptoms are hives typically accompanied by abdominal pain and mostly due to loss of discipline in eating and drinking. In other words, these hives are clearly associated with a food allergy. In some cases, there may even be intestinal parasites. The tongue coating is slimy and possibly yellow, while the pulse is slippery and rapid. The treatment principles are to dispel wind and discharge heat, disperse, lead away, and kill parasites. A commonly prescribed formula for this type of hives is *Fang Feng Tong Shen San* (Ledebouriella Communicate with the Sages Powder) with various modifications. Clearly in this pattern, it is important for the patient to eat a hypoallergenic, clear, bland diet. A simple Chinese herbal home remedy for both the wind heat and stomach and intestine damp heat patterns of hives is to make a tea out of cornsilk and Job's tears barley and drink 2 times each day for at least 10 days.

Common & plantar warts

Warts are a type of viral infection. Children are more prone to getting warts because of their weak immune systems in turn due to the inherent immaturity of their organs. In Chinese medicine, warts are called *qian ri chuang* or thousand day sores because they often spontaneously disappear after 1,000 days or so. In children, warts are due to a combination of factors. Usually there is a combination of damp heat brewing and steaming with blood deficiency in turn due to a weak spleen. This damp heat causes obstruction to the flow of qi and blood which accumulates to form the wart. Because there is an accumulation of tissue, there is also an element of phlegm nodulation. Because the top of the wart is dry and scaly, there is typically an element of blood dryness and deficiency. If the wart is kept covered and becomes damp, it often becomes inflamed due to this aggravating the underlying damp heat. Likewise, if the wart is picked at by the child, it will easily become inflamed also due to the underlying damp heat.

In Chinese medicine, the treatments for warts are very similar to their modern Western medical counterparts. Either caustic herbs are applied on top of the wart in order to chemically burn it off or moxibustion is used to physically burn it off. Frankly, if and when warts need to come off, one should go to a Western MD to have them removed. For this kind of thing, Western medicine is safer, quicker, and more efficient.

Poison ivy

Strictly speaking, poison ivy, which is a kind of contact dermatitis or inflammation of the skin, is not a pediatric disease. But kids being kids, they often go out to play in wooded areas, and kids being kids, they are not always knowledgeable or careful about what plants they come in contact with. In Chinese medicine, because the skin lesions caused by poison ivy and poison oak are red, hot, painful, itchy, and weep a watery fluid when the blisters break, they are seen as a type of damp heat condition. In the West, poison ivy is treated primarily by the topical application of calamine lotion, and calamina is also a topical ingredient for external application in Chinese medicine as well. However, in Chinese medicine there are also internal herbal decoctions which can be taken to more quickly reduce the itching, inflammation, and discomfort. For instance, modified versions of *Er Miao San* (Two Wonders Powder) may be prescribed. At the same time there are Chinese herbal washes, such as *Ku Shen Tang* (Sophora Decoction) that can be applied locally instead of such things as calamine lotion.

Nosebleed

It is not uncommon for children to develop nosebleeds for no apparent reason. Usually parents pay little or no attention to this unless the nosebleeds are frequent and severe. Nevertheless, although such nosebleeds are not life-threatening, they can give a clue about the constitutional imbalance of the child and, therefore, can help identify a better diet. In Chinese pediatrics, there are two main patterns of children's nosebleed. These are lung heat combined with an external invasion, and spleen/stomach brewing or smoldering heat.

In the first pattern, there is a tendency for the lungs to already or habitually harbor heat. If the child then "catches cold" or is invaded by an external pathogen, this adds even more heat to the lungs and this heat causes the blood to boil over like milk on a stove allowed to boil too quickly. Although this metaphor seems extreme, it says nothing about severity. It only graphically describes how Chinese medicine says heat causes abnormal bleeding. The symptoms of this pattern are headache, aversion to wind, a dry mouth and nose, occasional bloody nose, cough with scanty phlegm, and a floating rapid pulse. The treatment principles are to clear heat and resolve the exterior, cool the blood and stop bleeding. The formula used may be similar to *Qing Liang Zhi Nu Tang*

(Clear & Cool Stop Nosebleed Decoction). Obviously, children with a tendency to this pattern of nosebleeds need to avoid hot, spicy foods which aggravate heat.

The second pattern of pediatric nosebleed has to due primarily with diet. Because of overeating hot, spicy foods, and greasy, fried, fatty foods, heat has accumulated and is brewing in the spleen and stomach. This heat causes the blood to boil over, resulting in nosebleed. The symptoms of this pattern are blood occasionally flowing from the nose, dry nose, bad breath, thirst and a preference for cold drinks, constipation, a yellow tongue coating, and a slippery, rapid pulse. The treatment principles are to clear the stomach and to downbear fire. *Bai Hu Tang* (White Tiger Decoction) with various modifications is usually the formula chosen to treat this pattern of pediatric nosebleed. Children with this pattern need to stay away from hot, spicy and greasy, fatty foods. Parenthetically, I myself have this pattern and I will get a runny nose if I eat something extremely hot and spicy. Because this pattern is also associated with constipation, canker sores, and other similar problems, keeping the bowels open and freely flowing is very important. When children with this pattern get sick, they tend to develop a fever quickly.

Canker sores

Canker sores refer to small sores on the gums and the inner walls of the cheeks. Children tend to get these from time to time. They rarely require any kind of medical attention and the child may make no mention of them. Mostly they are due to damp heat smoldering in the spleen and stomach, similar to the second pattern of nosebleed above. Avoidance of hot, spicy foods and greasy, fatty foods is usually important in this kind of pattern as is keeping the bowel movements open and free flowing. If the canker sores require treatment or there are canker sores along with some other complaint, usually some modification of *Bai Hu Tang* (White Tiger Decoction) or *Gan Lu Yin* (Sweet Dew Drink) will clear heat and disinhibit dampness, thus restoring balance to the organism. A Chinese home herbal remedy for treating canker sores is to boil 5g of fresh peppermint in 1 cup of water and add a little salt. Drink this as a tea frequently through the day. This can also help toothache and nosebleed due to heat in the stomach.

Another herbal home remedy is to boil watercress and carrots into a soup and drink. For better results, a few senna leaves are added. Senna is usually available at Western health food stores. Senna is a laxative herb, and this shows that constipation due to heat in the stomach and intestines can also be associated with canker sores.

Conjunctivitis

Conjunctivitis is also referred to as pink eye, especially in children. It is not listed as a pediatric disease in Chinese pediatric texts but because children often develop this condition, I have included it for the sake of parents who may not know otherwise what to do about pink eye. Acute conjunctivitis means an acute inflammation of the conjunctiva of the eye. According to Western medicine, this may be due to viruses, bacteria, or allergies. In Chinese medicine, redness is associated with some sort of pathological heat in the body. There are five main patterns associated with conjunctivitis. These are an external invasion of wind heat, heat toxins, stomach heat hyperactive above, liver fire hyperactive above, and yin deficiency with internal heat. In children, the two most commonly encountered patterns are the wind heat external invasion and the stomach heat hyperactive above.

We have already discussed the signs and symptoms of wind heat above under several other diseases. Stomach heat causes conjunctivitis because the stomach channel connects directly with the eye. Symptoms of stomach heat include frequent hunger, a desire for cold drinks, possible constipation or diarrhea, restlessness, a red tongue with a yellow coating, and a slippery, rapid pulse. The treatment for stomach heat conjunctivitis is to drain the stomach and clear heat. One prescription that can be used to treat conjunctivitis due to stomach heat is *Xie Xin Tang* (Drain the Heart Decoction) with modifications. However, because wind heat can stir up and aggravate stomach heat, often these two mechanisms occur together in children, thus producing conjunctivitis. A simple Chinese herbal home remedy for conjunctivitis due to stomach heat is to make a tea out of broccoli and carrot, both of which are cool by nature. Another possibility is to make tea out of chrysanthemum flowers (Flos Chrysanthemi Morifolii, *Ju Hua*) which are available from Oriental specialty food shops and Chinese apothecaries. A variation of this remedy is to make a tea out of both chrysanthemum flowers and spinach. Further, the warm chrysanthemum flowers used to make this tea can be placed over the affected eye as a type of poultice. Yet another possibility is to make a tea out of whole dandelions. And finally, one can grate cucumbers and make a poultice to apply to the affected eye.

Hyperactivity

In Chinese medicine, pediatric hyperactivity has to do with the Chinese concept of the spirit residing in the heart. Spirit here refers to the mind and to consciousness. If the spirit is healthy, then it is calm. If the spirit is calm, then the mind is not agitated nor the body restless. According to Chinese medicine, there are three basic causes which can disturb the spirit residing in the heart — either the spirit is not nourished sufficiently which causes the spirit to flutter around nervously, some sort of heat wafts upward and disturbs the spirit as if one's house were on fire, or phlegm blocks the portals or openings of the heart. In this latter case, the spirit's connection with the outside world is confused and hindered as if shutters had been put on all the doors and windows of the mind's house. Each of these three basic mechanisms of a disturbed heart spirit becomes the basis for one of the three TCM patterns which describe pediatric hyperactivity.

The first of these three patterns is heart/spleen insufficiency. In this case there is not enough qi and blood to nourish the spirit. Thus the spirit becomes nervous due to lack of sufficient nourishment. The symptoms of this pattern are a sallow yellow or dull white facial complexion, pale nails and lips, fatigue, insomnia, heart palpitations, shortness of breath, a poor appetite, a tendency to loose stools, poor memory, a fat, pale tongue with a thin, white coating, and a fine, weak pulse. The treatment principles for this pattern are to strengthen the spleen and supplement the heart, supplement the qi and nourish the blood. One commonly used Chinese herbal formula for treating this pattern of pediatric hyperactivity is *Yang Xin Yi Pi Tang* (Nourish the Heart & Boost the Spleen Decoction) with modifications. In addition, the diet should be a nourishing, cooked, warm, clear, bland diet. By nourishing, I mean that there should be a little more animal protein in this child's diet in order to help manufacture sufficient blood. Soups made out of black beans, chicken or beef broth, and lots of root and leafy green vegetables are good. Acupuncture is not such an effective treatment method for this pattern of hyperactivity.

The second pattern is yin deficiency, yang hyperactivity. This child is usually thin and highly strung. In Chinese medicine, yin refers to the substance of the body as well as nourishing blood and body fluids. When healthy and abundant, this yin keeps yang in check. Yang refers to function and activity, movement and change. It also is associated with warmth and heat in the body. If yin is insufficient, due to a constitutional yin deficiency or over-consumption of yin by lack of adequate sleep, prolonged emotional stress, or drug use, than yang becomes hyperactive and heat tends to flush upward to disturb the heart spirit. Besides tending to be thin, children with this pattern also have a red tongue with scanty coating or a pale tongue with a red tip. Their pulses are fine and rapid and they tend to suffer from insomnia, heart palpitations, agitation, dizziness, ringing in the ears, possible low back pain, possible bed-wetting at night, flushed cheeks, and possible night sweats. The treatment principles are to supplement the kidneys and enrich yin, subdue yang and quiet the spirit. Your practitioner may choose a formula such as *You Yin Qian Yang Wan* (Foster Yin & Subdue Yang Pills) with modifications for this purpose. Usually this pattern requires herbal supplementation and takes longer to show results that the preceding pattern.

The third pattern of pediatric hyperactivity is actually a mixture of phlegm blocking or confounding the portals of the heart, and heat disturbing the heart spirit. Its signs and symptoms are easy anger or pronounced irritability, vexation and restlessness, possible nausea, possible excessive phlegm, a stuffy chest or feeling like the chest is oppressed, a bitter taste in the mouth when waking up in the morning, a tongue with red edges and a slimy, yellow coating, and a wiry, slippery, rapid pulse. The treatment principles are to clear heat and transform phlegm while regulating the flow of qi. For this pattern, professional practitioners of Chinese medicine often prescribe *Huang Lian Wen Dan Tang* (Coptis Warm the Gallbladder Decoction) with various modifications. This is an extremely effective formula when patients have this pattern and results come with almost startling rapidity. Because this pattern is complicated by phlegm and the spleen is the root of phlegm production, it is vitally important to avoid foods which either weaken the spleen, such as chilled, cold, raw foods or sugar and sweets, or foods which cause dampness and phlegm to be generated in the body, such as sugar and sweets, dairy foods, and fatty, greasy, fried foods. Because this pattern is, in part, due to poor flow of qi in turn due to emotional stress and because acupuncture can help move the qi and free its flow, acupuncture for this pattern can be a useful adjunctive or supplementary treatment.

Measles

Measles, also called rubeola, is an acute, epidemic, infectious disease caused by the measles virus. It may strike at any age during childhood, and it may attack adults who have never had measles before. It mainly occurs during the spring. Once one has had measles, they then have a life-time immunity. In the past, measles were often a life-threatening disease, especially for children. Fortunately, because of hereditary immunity built up over generations among most Westerners, measles is rarely fatal these days.

In Chinese medicine, measles is believed to be due to a combination of *tai du* or fetal toxins plus invasion by an external pathogen. In other words, there is a predisposing factor to measles and that is this concept of fetal toxins. Fetal toxins are toxins developed during pregnancy. Not every person develops the same kind or amount of fetal toxins. Some children, due to the mother's diet and lifestyle or due to the mother's health at the time of conception and during pregnancy, inherit or develop more fetal toxins than others. For instance, if the mother recently had a severe, acute febrile disease just before conception or during pregnancy, this may predispose the child to more fetal toxins. Or if the mother had a very bad diet, eating lots of greasy, fried, fatty foods and drinking lots of alcohol, this might also result in the accumulation of more fetal toxins. Once generated, these toxins lie dormant in the body until they are provoked by some external factor. Thus they are also referred to as *fu wen xie* or deep-lying warm evils.

Chinese medicine divides the progression of measles into two basic types and three basic stages. First of all, there are those cases of measles that follow the normal progression of this disease and those that follow an abnormal progression. Basically, Chinese doctors want to see the measles rash "come out" fully on the body. This is then taken for a sign that the righteous or healthy energy of the body is sufficient to fight the evil or disease energy and that, in fact, the righteous energy is kicking this evil energy out of the body. Since this evil energy was generated during pregnancy, once it is gone, it is gone for good. If, on the other hand, the righteous energy of the body is not sufficiently strong to kick these toxins out of the body, then they sink back into the body and can cause a variety of diseases at a later date.

The following chart gives some idea about the healthy or correct progression of this disease and an abnormal or unhealthy progression.

	Favorable symptoms			Unfavorable symptoms
Stage	Before rash appears	Rash appears	Rash fades	
Fever	Chills & fever	Continuous fever	Fever subsides	Fever too high or not high enough; high fever does not abate in the last stage
Cough	Mild	Worse	Better	Persistent, severe cough, shortness of breath, flaring of the wings of the nose
Spirit	Normal	Restless	Normal	Restlessness, mental cloudiness, delirium
Sweating	Mild	Mild	Mild	No sweating, dry heat sensation of the skin or profuse sweating with cold limbs
Order of eruption	Hairlines behind ear, neck, face, back, chest, four limbs, nose, hands, feet			Delayed eruption or untimely fading of rash
Distribution	Even			Sparse and indistinct or dense and joining up into larger areas; absence of rash on the face and nose in severe cases
Color	Bright red and moist-looking			Pale and dull or dark purple

In the pre-eruption stage, as long as the disease is progressing normally, the symptoms are usually a mild cough, watery, red eyes and photophobia, puffy, swollen eyelids, mental dullness and a wan, dispirited affect, possibly vomiting and diarrhea, a sore throat, greyish white spots in the mouth with red border, known as Koplik's spots, a thin, white or thin, yellow tongue coating, and a floating rapid pulse. These symptoms mostly correspond to the two Chinese organs of the lungs and spleen. The treatment principles are to use acrid, cool medicinals to out-thrust the exterior or, in other words, promote the expression of the rash. One of the most commonly used formulas for this purpose is *Sheng Ma Ge Gen Tang* (Cimicifuga & Pueraria Decoction) with modifications. This is essentially a wind heat pattern with spleen complications. Therefore, one should not use cold bath or cold water sponge baths to try to bring down the fever. Such an external application of cold would only close the skin firmly shut, thus preventing the expulsion of the rash.

In order to help the rash express itself quickly and completely, there are several Chinese herbal home remedies. First, one can boil 250-500g of fresh coriander (also called cilantro or Chinese parsley at many grocery stores in the United States). After allowing this to cool, one can wash the upper body with this simple and thin, white or thin, yellow tongue coating, and a floating rapid pulse. these symptoms mostly correspond to the two Chinese organs of the lungs and spleen. The treatment readily available herbal decoction. Secondly, one can crush 5g of sunflower seeds and make these into tea. Drink this tea two times each day. Third, cook carrots, parsley, and water chestnuts together and eat. Or fourth, one can boil 9g of cherry seeds in 1 cup of water and drink the liquid. At the same time, boil 150g of cherry seeds in 4 cups of water and use the liquid to bathe the body.

In the eruption stage, the symptoms are usually a high fever which does not abate, thirst with a desire to drink, severe cough, a continued dull affect, gummed up eyes, irritability and restlessness, possible delirium during high fever, possible twitching or convulsions due to high fever, a raised, red maculopapular rash starting first behind the ears and then spreading to the neck, face, head, chest, back, and limbs. The rash is bright red in color and may exude a watery fluid. Later the rash spreads and joins into larger areas and its color becomes darker. The tongue is red with a yellow coating, and the pulse is surging and rapid. The treatment principles in this stage are to clear heat, resolve toxins, and out-thrust the rash. A commonly prescribed formula for this stage is _Qing Jie Tou Biao Tang_ (Clear, Resolve & Out-thrust the Exterior Decoction) with additions and subtractions.

During this high fever stage, if there is delirium, an acupuncturist should be called in order to let a drop or two of blood from several points. In part, the signs and symptoms of this stage have to do with evil or pathogenic heat having entered the blood which then disturbs the heart spirit which is nourished by the blood. Letting a drop or two of blood from certain points helps clear this heat from the blood and can bring down the fever.

In stage three, called the fading of the rash, the symptoms are that the rash gradually diminishes. The skin becomes flaky and scaly and gradually returns to a normal color within 7-10 days. The high fever diminishes, the spirit recovers, digestion and appetite improve day by day, and the cough gets less and less until it disappears. The tongue is red with scanty fluids and scanty coating, while the pulse is fine and soft or fine and rapid. These symptoms correspond to a yin deficiency pattern where yin fluids have been consumed and exhausted by the prolonged high fever. The treatment principles are to support the righteous and nourish yin while simultaneously clearing any remaining heat. Professional practitioners of Chinese medicine will often prescribe _Sha Shen Mai Dong Tang_ (Glehnia & Ophiopogon Decoction) with modifications for this pattern.

If the parent thinks that the measles are not progressing normally, they should definitely seek the advice and aid of a professionally trained practitioner of Chinese medicine. Chinese medicine identifies a number of different patterns of measles not progressing normally and has treatments for each of these patterns. Chinese medicine is also very effective for treating any sequelae, _i.e._, left-over, after effects from the measles, such as continuing, low-grade, tidal fevers in the evenings, night sweats, constipation, lack of appetite, diarrhea, fatigue, night terrors, or patches of dry, itchy skin, boils, or ulcers.

Traditionally, parents would hold measles parties so that children would become infected when they were still young. In other words, if a child came down with a case of measles, parents of other children would bring those children to the house of the infected child specifically so that their children would catch the measles too. The idea is that it is better for children to get this disease when they are still young and to get it out of the way, and there is some sense to this practice since this disease is often worse in older patients.

Rubella

We used to call rubella German measles when I was a kid. Rubella is a mild infectious disease marked by mild fever, cough, and a sand-like, light red rash which appears and then fades quickly. According to Western medicine, it is due to a virus. It most commonly affects children under five years of age and most commonly occurs in the winter and spring. In Chinese medicine, rubella is seen as a wind heat invasion of the lungs and defensive level of the qi. (When diagnosing and treating acute, infectious diseases, Chinese doctors sometimes describe the depth of the invading pathogen. The defensive level is the most superficial. This is then followed by the qi level, constructive level, and blood level respectively.) It is sometimes further divided into a mild condition and a heavier condition with more prevalent heat.

The symptoms of the mild condition are fever, aversion to wind, cough, runny nose, a rash over the entire body for 1-2 days which is pale red or bright red in color and is accompanied by an itching sensation, and a floating, moderately rapid pulse. The treatment principles of this pattern are to course wind and clear heat. Representative Chinese herbal formulas for treating this condition are modifications of *Yin Qiao San* (Lonicera & Forsythia Powder) and *Jia Wei Xiao Du Yin* (Added Flavors Disperse Toxins Drink).

The heavier condition is characterized by more heat. Its symptoms are a moderately high fever, a bright red colored rash whose spots are somewhat densely packed,

140

irritability, thirst, yellowish, scanty urine, and relatively red lips and tongue. The pulse is still floating but more rapid than in the preceding pattern. The treatment principles are to clear heat and cool the blood, and commonly prescribed formulas include *Qiao He Tang* (Forsythia & Mint Decoction) and *Tou Zhen Liang Jie Tang* (Out-thrust the Rash, Cooling & Resolving Decoction) with modifications.

Usually rubella is a mild disease and recovery is rapid and uncomplicated. It is better for a child to catch this disease when still young. If a woman catches this disease during the early stage of pregnancy, it can cause birth defects. Therefore, especially if one's child is a girl, if one does not intend to immunize against this disease, then a German measles party is a good idea.

Chickenpox

Chickenpox is also known as varicella. It too is an acute, epidemic, viral infection which is very common in young children. Children under 15 years of age are the most susceptible and it mostly occurs in the winter and spring. It is a highly communicable disease and its symptoms are usually mild with a favorable and complete recovery. The Chinese name for this disease is *shui dou* or water pox, since it is characterized by the eruption of watery blisters all over the body. Like rubella, Chinese medicine divides most cases of chickenpox into two basic patterns.

The first pattern is called wind heat mixed with dampness. Its symptoms are fever, headache, stuffy nose, runny nose, cough, and a moist, red rash made up of water blisters filled with a clear fluid. These blisters appear first on the scalp, face, and torso. Urination and defecation are normal, the tongue has a thin, white coating, and the pulse is floating and rapid. This is once again a wind heat invasion of the lungs and exterior part of the body. However, because there are water-filled blisters, Chinese medicine says that there is an element of dampness as well. The treatment principles are, therefore, to course wind, clear heat, and seep dampness. The most commonly used Chinese herbal formula for these purposes is *Yin Qiao San* (Lonicera & Forsythia Powder) with modifications. We have seen this formula recommended under several different diseases above when the pattern is wind heat. This is a very good example of how TCM bases its treatment on pattern discrimination and how different diseases often receive the same treatment *if the pattern is the same.*

The second pattern is internal heat flaming and exuberance. It is characterized by strong fever, vexation and agitation, a dry mouth and red lips, red cheeks and face, scanty, yellowish urine, large pox which are densely packed and which are colored purplish and dark and are filled with a turbid fluid, a scarlet tongue with a thick, yellow, dry coating, and a surging, rapid pulse. The treatment principles for this pattern are to clear heat, resolve toxins, and seep dampness. Representative Chinese herbal formulas are *Qing Li Jie Du Tang* (Clear the Interior & Resolve Toxins Decoction) and *Qing Ying Tang* (Clear the Constructive Decoction) with various modifications depending on the signs and symptoms of the individual child.

Because this is a damp heat condition, a soup or dilute porridge made out of mung beans can be helpful, and certainly the child should not be allowed to eat any hot, spicy or greasy, fatty foods. That means chips and salsa is out, as is chocolate. The child should be kept from scratching the pustules as much as possible since this can cause scarring and even infection. If the pustules are oozing or if there is danger of infection, professional practitioners of Chinese medicine can prescribe various herbal washes for external application to the lesions.

Scarlatina

We have talked briefly about scarlatina or scarlet fever above under strep throat. Scarlatina is another acute, infectious disease marked by fever, swelling, sore throat, and a diffuse, bright red skin rash all over the body. However, unlike the several preceding diseases which are due to viruses of one sort or another, scarlatina is a bacterial infection. It, like so many other acute, infectious diseases, is most common in the winter and spring, and it commonly affects children between 2-8 years of age.

Chinese medicine divides scarlet fever into three main patterns. The first of these is evils assailing and entering the lungs and defensive. Its symptoms are fever which goes from low to high, slight aversion to chill, thirst, headache, cough, sore throat, flushed red skin, an indistinct, bright red rash, a red tongue with a thin, white coating, and a floating, rapid pulse. Its treatment principles are to diffuse the lungs and out-thrust the rash by using acrid, cool herbs and to clear heat and disinhibit or ease the throat. Once again, *Yin Qiao San* (Lonicera & Forsythia Powder) with modifications is the formula most commonly chosen by professional practitioners of Chinese medicine to treat this pattern, however with the addition of ingredients specifically to promote the complete eruption of the rash.

The second pattern is toxic evils entering the qi and constructive levels. This is characterized by high fever, a flushed, red face, thirst with a desire to drink, swelling, pain, and erosion of the throat, a densely pack, bright red or purple rash, dry stools, scanty, reddish yellow urine, a dark red tongue with thorns, and a deep yellow, coarse tongue coating, and a rapid, forceful pulse. The treatment principles for dealing with this pattern of scarlet fever are to clear the qi level and cool the constructive level, drain fire and resolve toxins. A representative Chinese herbal formula for this pattern is *Liang Ying Qing Pi Tang* (Cool the Constructive & Clear the Qi Decoction) with modifications.

If the high fever has gone on for some time, this may consume and exhaust the healthy yin fluids of the body. Therefore, towards the tail end or recuperative phase of this disease, one may see the third pattern commonly associated with scarlatina emerge. This is a yin deficiency pattern with lingering heat. Its signs and symptoms are gradual diminishing of high fever and skin rash, dry skin with scaling and peeling, diminished sore throat, thirst, dry lips, dry cough, a red tongue with scanty fluids, and a fine, rapid pulse. The treatment principles for this pattern are to nourish yin and generate fluids, clear heat and moisten the throat. Above we have seen *Sha Shen Mai Dong Tang* (Glehnia & Ophiopogon Decoction) with modifications used to treat the recuperative stage of other febrile diseases, and here it can be used again. In terms of foods which can help moisten dryness and generate fluids, one can eat cooked pears, applesauce, and a little sugar and warm, boiled milk.

Because scarlet fever can be a scary and dangerous disease if not adequately treated, daily acupuncture can be done to help clear heat and drain fire. My own son has had scarlet fever which was not treated by antibiotics but only by Chinese herbs. Eventually, all the skin on his palms and soles of his feet peeled. He never had any problems with heart palpitations or other rheumatic complications of the heart. In other words, although antibiotics may be considered in the case of scarlatina, they are not mandatory and Chinese medicine can be used to treat this disease.

Mumps

Mumps are technically referred to as epidemic parotitis which simply means an epidemic inflammation of the parotid glands in the throat. Mumps are a type of viral infection which can attack a person at any age but which is usually far less serious and uncomfortable as a child than as a grown-up. Like many other viral contagions, once one has had mumps one usually has a lifetime immunity, though it is possible for a few people to develop them a second time. Winter and spring are again the most likely seasons to contract this disease. In Chinese medicine, inflamed, painful swellings are often associated with the concept of toxins. Toxins are usually warm or hot, although not always. Toxins tend to cause very painful, swollen, red, and oftentimes pussy, purulent conditions. Therefore, TCM divides mumps into two main patterns — heat toxins in the exterior of the body and heat toxins in the interior of the body.

The symptoms of heat toxins in the exterior of the body are mild fever, mild aversion to chill, swelling and pain of the parotid region on one or both sides of the throat under the jaw, difficulty swallowing, a red, sore throat, a red tongue with a thin, white or slightly yellow coating, and a floating, rapid pulse. The treatment principles are to dispel wind and clear heat, scatter nodulation and disperse swelling. The Chinese herbal formula frequently used for these purposes by professional practitioners of Chinese medicine is again *Yin Qiao San* (Lonicera & Forsythia Powder) with modifications.

The symptoms of heat toxins in the interior of the body are high fever, headache, thirst with a desire to drink, possible vomiting, swelling and distention of the parotid glands which feel hard to the touch and painful when pressed, redness, swelling, and sore throat, a red tongue with a yellow coating, and a slippery, rapid pulse. The treatment principles for this pattern of epidemic parotitis are to clear heat and resolve toxins, soften the hard and disperse swelling. *Pu Ji Xiao Du Yin* (Dispersing Toxins Drink [from the book *Universal Relief]*) with modifications is a good choice of a guiding prescription for this condition.

Because both these patterns are heat patterns, the patient should avoid eating anything greasy or fatty or hot and spicy. Chinese folk remedies for mumps include boiling 20g of dried lily flower (available at Oriental specialty food stores) and drinking as a soup after adding some salt to taste. As for external applications, there are a number of these in Chinese medicine. One is to crush 10g of peeled garlic in 10ml of rice vinegar and then apply this externally to the swollen gland(s). Another is to crush a potato and squeeze out the juice. Mix this juice with vinegar and apply this locally. One can also grind 50-70 aduki beans into a powder. Mix this with warm water and egg white or with honey to make into a paste. Apply this paste over the affected glands and cover with a gauze bandage. Further, one can pound either fresh hibiscus leaves or fresh portulaca into a paste and apply this over the swollen glands. The portulaca that is used is the common purslane that grows as a weed in gardens and in sidewalk cracks. It is also possible to use acupuncture to help relieve the pain in the throat and quicken the resolution of the disease.

And finally, to reduce the pain and swelling of swollen glands (from mumps and other sources), one can use alternating hot and cold compresses. Begin by thoroughly wetting a towel with hot water. Wring out the towel so that it does not drip and wrap this around the child's throat being sure that it covers the swollen glands. Cover this wet towel with a dry one to both keep in the heat and prevent dripping. Be sure that the rest of the child's body is covered by a blanket in order to prevent chilling. Leave this warm compress in place for 15 minutes. Then remove and replace with a towel that has been run under very cold water. Leave this in place for five minutes, covered the same way as

145

the hot compress. Again replace this cold compress with a hot compress and leave in place for 15 minutes. This can be repeated one, two, or three times each day to provide relief from pain and to help speed up the course of recovery.

Once glands get swollen and hard, they do not go down that quickly. Therefore, parents should not get worried if the glands are still relatively large and hard after all the other symptoms have disappeared. In adults, mumps can involve the testes in men and the breasts in women, but these complications rarely occur in children.

Diphtheria

Diphtheria is an acute, bacterial, upper respiratory tract infection. It is characterized by the formation of greyish white membranes over the mucus membranes of the pharynx, larynx, and nose. This is accompanied by fever, sore throat, and cough with noisy inhalation. Although this disease may occur in any season of the year, it is most prevalent in the fall and winter, and children under 10 years of age are most susceptible. Furthermore, the younger the child, the more severe this disease tends to be. Even though this disease is not a common one in the West, because a growing number of parents are choosing not to immunize their children against it, I have chosen to say something about its Chinese treatment in this book. Nonetheless, any child suspected of having diphtheria should be under the care of a Western MD as well as any care given by a practitioner of Chinese medicine. Diphtheria can be a life-threatening disease.

In Chinese medicine, diphtheria is categorized as a seasonal, pestilential disease due to invasion by a particularly virulent hot pathogenic qi. Its treatment in Chinese medicine is based on the discrimination of three basic patterns. The first pattern is wind heat. Its symptoms are a mild fever, an inflamed, swollen, sore throat, greyish white spot-like membranes covering the back of the throat which are difficult to scrape off, difficulty swallowing, a red-tipped tongue with a thin, white coating, and a floating, rapid pulse. The treatment principles are to dispel wind, clear heat, and resolve toxins, and once again, *Yin Qiao San* (Lonicera & Forsythia Powder) with modifications is the usual formula of choice for this pattern.

The second pattern is yin deficiency with internal heat. Its symptoms are an inflamed, swollen throat with greyish yellow stripe-like membranes spreading over the uvula (the little tab of skin which hangs down at the back of the throat) and upper palate, dry mouth and throat, fever, cough, a hoarse voice, bad breath, a dark red tongue with scanty fluids and a scanty, yellow coating, and a fine, rapid pulse. The treatment principles for this pattern are to nourish yin, clear heat, and resolve toxins. Professional practitioners of Chinese medicine often use formulas such as *Yang Yin Qing Fei Tang* (Nourish Yin & Clear the Lungs Decoction) with modifications for this pattern of diphtheria.

And the third pattern commonly associated with diphtheria is diphtheria due to pestilential evils. As stated above, pestilential evils suggest an extreme type of toxic, hot pathogen. Therefore, the symptoms of this pattern are a very severe sore throat, the grey membrane spreading to and beyond the tonsils, swelling of the neck, cough, a hoarse voice, noisy inhalation, difficulty breathing, restlessness, and cyanosis of the lips. The tongue is red with a thick, yellow coating, and the pulse is slippery and rapid. This pattern describes a very severe stage of diphtheria. Its treatment principles are to disinhibit or clear heat and resolve toxins, transform phlegm and disinhibit or ease the throat. A common representative formula often used in the TCM treatment of this pattern of diphtheria is *Shen Xian Huo Ming Yin* (Spirit Immortal Rescue Life Drink) with modifications depending upon the exact signs and symptoms of the patient. In addition, bleeding several points near the fingertips with acupuncture can help bring down the fever and reduce the pain and swelling of the throat.

A simple Chinese herbal home remedy for diphtheria is to drink a tea made out of carrot tops. However, one should not think that this is a sufficient treatment for such a potentially serious and life-threatening disease. It is merely offered here as an adjunctive or supporting treatment when drunk as a background beverage or tea.

Traumatic injuries

As mentioned above, kids will be kids. That means that a certain amount of cuts and bruises, and burns and stings are part of the process of growing up. Children's coordination is not mature, nor is their assessment of what is safe. Therefore, although Chinese pediatric texts do not say anything about traumatic injuries, Western parents would, I believe, be disappointed and frustrated if I left this topic unaddressed.

Burns

There are a number of very simple Chinese herbal home remedies for burns. These include putting either fresh carrot juice, fresh cucumber juice, fresh potato juice, fresh aloe juice, fresh ginger juice, or honey to the burn itself. One can also apply roasted sesame oil or ground sesame seeds, *i.e., tahini.*

Although I have generally cautioned against using Asian-manufactured patent or ready-made medicines, there are a number of safe and effective Oriental patent medicines for external and firstaid use in the case of traumatic injuries. In the case of traumatic injuries, one typically needs a treatment which is ready right now. Since most of these medicines are not taken internally, their use is safe and warranted. One such Chinese patent medicine for burns is Ching Wan Burn Ointment. This is the single best burn ointment I know. It is available at Chinese apothecaries in China towns in major Western cities.

Bruises

A bruise or contusion is a closed wound typically due to being struck or in a fall. Bruises cause a black and blue mark which, in Chinese medicine, is static blood which has pooled outside the blood vessels due to the strike or fall causing the local blood vessels to break or rupture. The Chinese medical treatment principles for dealing with bruises are, therefore, to move the blood and dispel stasis. Two effective Chinese patent medicines for external application to bruises and contusions are Tieh Ta Yao Gin and Wan Hua Oil.

Cuts

In order to stop bleeding, one can sprinkle carbonized human hair into the wound. To make this, place some hair clippings into a cast iron lidded pot and put in an oven to cook. This will cause a very bad, sulphurous smell; so be sure you do this with the windows and doors open. After the hair has carbonized in the bottom of the pot, allow it to cool, remove, and powder finely. Then store in a clean, dry, lidded glass jar for use. One can also by Crinis Carbonisatus (*Xue Yu Tan*) at Chinese apothecaries. Another possibility is to sprinkle Alum (*Bai Fan*) into a cut or dry ginger powder. There is also the Chinese patent medicine, Yunnan Bai Yao. This powder can be sprinkled into a cut to stop bleeding. It also comes as capsules which can be taken internally to stop more serious bleeding. Alum and Yunnan Bai Yao are also available from Chinese apothecaries. Yet another possibility is to sprinkle powdered cuttlebone into the cut. Cuttlebone can be purchased at pet stores or at Chinese apothecaries under the name Os Sepiae Seu Sepiellae (*Hai Piao Xiao* or *Wu Zei Gu*).

If a cut becomes infected, as they sometimes do with children who have a propensity for playing in the dirt and for picking at scabs, then one can make a poultice of crushed burdock roots applied warm to the affected area. Burdock is a common weed growing widely throughout North America and it is also available as a food (sometimes under the Japanese name, *gobo*) at health food stores. Another possibility is to make a compress out of raw, crushed garlic. At the same time, drink 1 teacup of warm, boiled water mixed with 1 teacup of freshly squeezed *daikon* radish juice. Or powder some rhubarb root, available at Chinese apothecaries under the name Radix Et Rhizoma Rhei (*Da Huang* or *Chuan Jun*), mix with honey to form a thin paste, and apply locally.

Sprains & strains

When running and playing, it is not uncommon for children to twist their ankle or to strain a joint. Typically, our first response in the West is to ice such injuries. In Chinese medicine, ice may be applied for the first 24 hours, but after that, because the intense cold further restricts the flow of blood and such injuries in part involve already static blood, we do not recommend using ice after that. If the joint is still swollen, red, and inflamed, then one can make a poultice or plaster out of grated potato or grated taro root mixed with a little white flour to hold it together. This will help clear heat and thus eliminate inflammation as well as eliminate the dampness associated with the swelling and edema. Another possibility during the swollen, inflamed stage is to make a poultice out of crush tofu and a little white flour. Such poultices are applied to the affected area, which should be kept raised and immobile, and replaced every couple of hours.

If the sprain or strain is no longer hot to the touch or red to the sight but is still markedly swollen, then one can cook some buckwheat and mix that with white flour to make a poultice. Apply this to the swollen area in order to help eliminate the dampness and edema.

There are also so-called "hit pills" (*die da wan* or *tieh ta wan* depending on whether they are manufactured in the People's Republic of China or Hong Kong/Taiwan). These are large pills made from powdered herbs mixed with honey. They contain a number of ingredients in order to move the qi and blood, dispel stasis and stop pain. One pill or a part of a pill may be taken 1-2 times per day for serious strains, sprains, contusions, and even dislocations and broken bones *as long as there is no marked bleeding*. In addition, there are a number of commercially available Chinese herbal liniments, plasters, soaks, and compresses. These can be purchased at a Chinese apothecary or from a professional practitioner of Chinese medicine. Parents of active children may find it useful to keep a selection of these kinds of ready-made medicines in a Chinese herbal first aid kit. A simple home liniment for external application can be made by boiling some safflowers in some vinegar. Then strain out the safflowers and bottle this for later use.

Imbedded foreign objects

If one gets a thorn or splinter or some other, *small* foreign object imbedded in the skin, one can draw this out by taking a half of an onion and roasting it in an oven until soft. This is then applied over the object while still warm and kept in place for some time. Such a poultice of raw, roasted onion can help pull a foreign object from the skin.

Insect stings

A simple Chinese herbal home remedy for bee and other insect stings is to rub garlic juice into the site of injury. Another simple herbal remedy is to chew some tea leaves into a mash and then place this poultice on the site of the sting. And a third herbal home remedy is to make a taro root plaster with a pinch of salt and apply to the affected area.

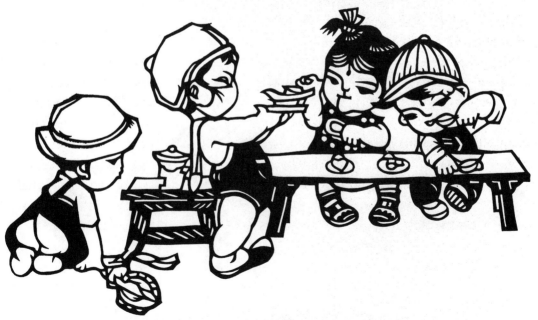

8
Case Histories

The following case histories give some idea how I treat infants and young children. As the reader will quickly discern, as a Chinese doctor, my main treatment modality is the prescription of Chinese herbal medicine taken internally. I rarely use acupuncture with children and infants. However, the reader should know that this is, to some extent, a stylistic preference on my part and, if you take your child to another practitioner, they may use acupuncture, laser acupuncture, magnetotherapy, or one or more of the other modalities of Chinese medicine.

Cough

Case 1: The patient was a 9 ½ month old little girl. Her main complaint was a wet cough. She had green mucus coming from her nose. She was waking a lot at night and was having trouble breathing at night. For some time she had been having only one bowel movement every three days which was typically hard and dry. However, the day of the visit the child's stools were loose and contained mucus. Her mother also said that she had begun teething two days before.

The wet cough meant that there was excessive phlegm in the lungs. The fact that the visible mucus was green meant that there was pathological heat in the lungs. The constipation and dry stools likewise suggested that she was overheated, thus drying out the stools. However, the presently loose stools with mucus suggested spleen deficiency with excessive phlegm and dampness. Therefore, the diagnosis I wrote down on the patient's chart was lung heat with spleen dampness. In this case, the appropriate treatment principles were to clear heat from the lungs while fortifying the spleen and to transform phlegm and eliminate dampness.

I wrote the child a Chinese herbal prescription which contained:

Rhizoma Anemarrhenae (*Zhi Mu*)
Bulbus Fritillariae (*Bei Mu*)
Rhizoma Pinelliae Ternatae (*Ban Xia*)
Sclerotium Poriae Cocos (*Fu Ling*)
Pericarpium Citri Reticulatae (*Chen Pi*)
Radix Scutellariae Baicalensis (*Huang Qin*)
Cortex Radicis Mori Albi (*Sang Bai Pi*)
Fructus Perillae Frutescentis (*Zi Su Zi*)
Radix Angelicae Dahuricae (*Bai Zhi*)

In this formula, the Anemarrhena, Scutellaria, and Cortex Mori all clear heat from the lungs and upper part of the body. Poria, Citrus, and Pinellia all strengthen the spleen and eliminate dampness, while Pinellia, Citrus, and Fritillaria transform phlegm. Fructus Perillae sends the lung qi downward and thus helps stop cough, and Angelica is a specific empirical remedy for green mucus coming from the nose. Thus each ingredient in this formula was chosen because its functions fulfilled one or more of the treatment principles or it relieves a specific symptom.

One packet of the above medicinals was given to the mother who was instructed to boil these in 2 cups of water down to 1 cup. She was then to give the child 2 droppers of this "tea" 4-6 times each day. I also counseled the mother on eliminating dairy products and sugars and sweets, including fruit juices, from the child's diet. Three days later, the mother called back to say that the herbs had been "perfect." The phlegm was now 90%

gone and the cough was almost nonexistent. At that point I told the mother to discontinue the herbs and the child was completely better in a day or two.

Case 2: The patient was an 8 month old little girl. She'd had a runny nose with yellow mucus for a couple of days. Recently she had developed a wet cough. Her mother said that she may be teething. There was no fever. The little girl was sleeping more than usual, her eyes were somewhat listless, and she had no appetite. Her extremities felt cold to the touch, which her mother said were always that way since she was born. There was a visible blue vein at the root of her nose between her two eyes. Thus my diagnosis was spleen deficiency, and heat and phlegm in the lungs. The phlegm was shown by the wet cough, the heat by the yellow mucus, and the spleen deficiency by the cold extremities, fatigue, lack of appetite, and listless eyes. Therefore, the treatment principles were to strengthen the spleen and supplement the qi, clear heat and transform phlegm. Although the diagnosis was similar in some regards to the previous patient's, in this case spleen deficiency was more evident. The prescription I wrote contained:

Sclerotium Poriae Cocos (*Fu Ling*)
Rhizoma Pinelliae Ternatae (*Ban Xia*)
Pericarpium Citri Reticulatae (*Chen Pi*)
Radix Codonopsis Pilosulae (*Dang Shen*)
Rhizoma Atractylodis Macrocephalae (*Bai Zhi*)
Radix Scutellariae Baicalensis (*Huang Qin*)
Semen Pruni Armeniacae (*Xing Ren*)
Fructus Perillae Frutescentis (*Zi Su Zi*)
Fructus Germinatus Oryzae Sativae (*Gu Ya*)
Corneum Endothelium Gigeriae Galli (*Ji Nei Jin*)

In this formula, Codonopsis, Atractylodes, and Poria all strengthen the spleen and supplement the qi. Pinellia, Armeniaca, Perilla, and Citrus transform phlegm and stop coughing. Scutellaria clears heat from the lungs. And Oryza and Corneum Endothelium

Gigeriae Galli help improve the appetite by eliminating any stagnant food in the stomach.

The patient's mother was instructed to make and administer this formula the same as for the preceding patient. I also instructed her on the importance of a clear, bland diet, no sugar or dairy products, no fruit juices and raw foods. Two days later the mother called back to say that the child was no longer fatigued, her hands and feet were warmer, her appetite had returned, and her cough and runny nose had cleared up.

Vomiting

Case 1: The child was a 2 month old little boy. He had been vomiting thick white mucus ever since he was born, one time every few days. For the past three weeks, he had been sounding very mucousy when he breathed. He was not colicky, but his stools were loose and watery. His mother said his urine was very pale, "amazingly clear." His appetite was reduced and he seemed fatigued. My diagnosis was vomiting due to a cold stomach. The white mucus, clear urine, fatigue, lack of appetite, and loose stools all pointed to a spleen deficiency cold type of vomiting with phlegm and dampness. Therefore, the treatment principles were to supplement the spleen and warm the middle, transform phlegm and stop vomiting. The formula I wrote consisted of:

Radix Panacis Ginseng (*Ren Shen*)
Rhizoma Atractylodis Macrocephalae (*Bai Zhu*)
Rhizoma Pinelliae Ternatae (*Ban Xia*)
mix-fried Radix Glycyrrhizae (*Gan Cao*)
dry Rhizoma Zingiberis (*Gan Jiang*)
Flos Caryophylli (*Ding Xiang*)
Fructus Evodiae Rutecarpae (*Wu Zhu Yu*)
Cortex Cinnamomi (*Rou Gui*)

These were prescribed and administered the same as above. Four days later the mother reported that the child was much better. He had stopped vomiting, his stools were more formed, and he seemed much more energetic. In this formula, Ginseng, Atractylodes, and Glycyrrhiza (Licorice) all strengthen the spleen and supplement the qi. Pinellia transforms phlegm and eliminates dampness. It also directs the qi downward and vomiting is a symptom of erroneously upward counterflowing qi. Zingiber (Ginger), Caryophyllum (Cloves) Evodia, and Cinnamon all warm the center or stomach and also all direct upwardly counterflowing qi downward.

Earache

Case 1: The child was a 6 year old boy. He'd had a bad cough for the preceding three days and now he had a bad earache. His tools were on the hard side and he had bad breath. His appetite was poor and he was fatigued. His tongue was red with a yellow coating and his pulse was slippery, full, and rapid. I diagnosed the earache as heat in the stomach and intestines counterflowing upward to accumulate in the ear. The treatment principles were, therefore, to clear heat from the lungs and stomach while supplementing the spleen. The formula I prescribed was a version of *Xiao Chai Hu Tang* (Minor Bupleurum Decoction):

Radix Bupleuri (*Chai Hu*)
Radix Scutellariae Baicalensis (*Huang Qin*)
Gypsum Fibrosum (*Shi Gao*)
Rhizoma Pinelliae Ternatae (*Ban Xia*)
Radix Codonopsis Pilosulae (*Dang Shen*)
mix-fried Radix Glycyrrhizae (*Gan Cao*)
Fructus Zizyphi Jujubae (*Da Zao*)
uncooked Rhizoma Zingiberis (*Sheng Jiang*)

At the same time I gave the mother some eardrops made from water, Alum (*Bai Fan*), Borax (*Peng Sha*), and Borneol (*Bing Pian*). In addition, I needled *Pian Li* (LI 6). This is the point which controls the connecting vessel linking the stomach and intestines to the inner ear. For even more pain relief, I explained how to do alternating hot and cold compresses on the ear. The next day the earache was gone and the cough cleared up in another two days, at which time the child was back to normal.

Case 2: The child was a 16 month old little boy. Nine months previously he had gotten his first ear infection. His pediatrician put him on antibiotics. Since then he had been on five different antibiotics. He would get an ear infection, take antibiotics, the ear infection would clear up, and it would come back again after 5 days to a week. At this point, the MD was recommending tubes in the ears. At the time I saw the child, his stools fluctuated between loose and normal. Sometimes he had asthmatic wheezing at night which was accompanied by cough and runny nose with the mucus ranging between being clear to yellow. He seemed paler than normal, a little puffy looking, and he had cold hands and feet. The day before seeing me, he had vomited a white, mucousy material. The vein at the base of his index finger was larger and more prominent than normal and was purple in color.

My diagnosis was spleen weakness with stagnant food and phlegm which periodically would transform into pathological heat. Because he did not have an earache at the time I saw this child, I prescribed a simple modification of *Xiao Chai Hu Tang* (Minor Bupleurum Decoction):

Radix Bupleuri (*Chai Hu*)
Radix Codonopsis Pilosulae (*Dang Shen*)
Rhizoma Pinelliae Ternatae (*Ban Xia*)
Radix Scutellariae Baicalensis (*Huang Qi*)
mix-fried Radix Glycyrrhizae (*Gan Cao*)
Fructus Zizyphi Jujubae (*Da Zao*)
uncooked Rhizoma Zingiberis (*Sheng Jiang*)
Massa Medica Fermentata (*Shen Qu*)

I told the mother to administer this formula to the child continuously for several months. I also gave her a long talk on proper diet. The child had been eating raw fruits and vegetables, cold fruit juices, cold milk, lots of bread, peanut butter, cheese, sugars and sweets, including ice cream and frozen yogurt — in other words, the full catastrophe. The mother said that it would be hard to change the child's diet so radically at this point, but she also said she would try. I told her that she could expect an earache as soon as the present course of antibiotics was finished and that, when that happened, she should not run to the MD but rather call me.

Several days later, she did call me as predicted. The child had started batting at his ears as soon as the antibiotics were finished. His stools were very loose and an orangy-yellow color. There was the sound of mucus in his throat when he breathed. I prescribed a different version of *Xiao Chai Hu Tang*:

Radix Bupleuri (*Chai Hu*)
Radix Panacis Ginseng (*Ren Shen*)
Radix Scutellariae Baicalensis (*Huang Qin*)
Rhizoma Pinellia Ternatae (*Ban Xia*)
mix-fried Radix Glycyrrhizae (*Gan Cao*)
Fructus Zizyphi Jujubae (*Da Zao*)
uncooked Rhizoma Zingiberis (*Sheng Jiang*)
Pericarpium Citri Reticulatae (*Chen Pi*)
Rhizoma Acori Graminei (*Shi Chang Pu*)
Radix Ligustici Wallichii (*Chuan Xiong*)
Radix Angelicae Dahuricae (*Bai Zhi*)

The addition of the Citrus was to eliminate dampness and transform phlegm. The Acorus was to transform phlegm and open the portals of the ear. Ligusticum was meant to guide the other herbs up to the side of the head and to help stop pain. While Angelica was meant to stop pain in the head and to clear heat and eliminate dampness in the head. In addition, I gave the child the same ear drops described in the previous case. Within a day the earache got better and the child went back to the original formula.

Three months later, the child has not had another earache. His facial color is rosier, his hands and feet are warmer, and he does not look so pale and puffy. His breathing is clear and he seems to have more energy.

Diarrhea

Case 1: The child was a 2 ½ month old little boy. His mother brought him in to see me because he had explosive diarrhea which was greenish in color and which contained mucus. In addition, he drooled constantly, had hiccups two times a day for 15 minutes to an hour each time, and was real fussy due to gas pains. Sometimes he would scream and, when he screamed, his face would become very red and he would sweat. Otherwise he had cool hands and feet. My diagnosis of this case was spleen deficiency contracting fright. This meant that there was spleen deficiency and dampness but that this was aggravated by fright affecting the relationship between his spleen and liver. The treatment principles were, therefore, to strengthen the spleen, relax the liver, and calm fright wind. The formula I wrote consisted of:

Radix Codonopsis Pilosulae (*Dang Shen*)
Rhizoma Atractylodis Macrocephalae (*Bai Zhu*)
Sclerotium Poriae Cocos (*Fu Ling*)
Radix Puerariae (*Ge Gen*)
Herba Agastachis Seu Pogostemi (*Huo Xiang*)
Semen Dolichoris Lablab (*Bian Dou*)
Radix Auklandiae Lappae (*Mu Xiang*)
dry Rhizoma Zingiberis (*Gan Jiang*)
Radix Albus Paeoniae Lactiflorae (*Bai Shao*)
Ramulus Uncariae Cum Uncis (*Gou Teng*)

This formula was made and administered the same as the others above. In this formula, Codonopsis, Atractylodes, Dolichos, Poria and dry Ginger strengthen the spleen. Agastaches eliminates dampness. Pueraria is empirically known to stop diarrhea.

Auklandia harmonizes the liver and spleen. Peony relaxes the liver and Uncaria settles liver wind and calms fright. One week later the mother called to say that the stools were now normal, the child had less colic, and that he was much happier overall.

Thrush

Case 1: The patient was a 6 week old little girl. She had thrush, gas, and cold hands and feet. Her nails were pale and the vein at the base of the index finger was fine and hardly visible. Although thrush is often due to dampness and heat, it may also be due to spleen deficiency. This is called deficiency pattern thrush and that is what this child's TCM pattern was. The treatment principles were to strengthen the spleen and eliminate dampness. The formula consisted of:

Radix Panacis Ginseng (*Ren Shen*)
Rhizoma Atractylodis Macrocephalae (*Bai Zhu*)
Sclerotium Poriae Cocos (*Fu Ling*)
Radix Puerariae (*Ge Gen*)
Radix Auklandiae Lappae (*Mu Xiang*)
Herba Agastachis Seu Pogostemi (*Huo Xiang*)
Radix Glycyrrhizae (*Gan Cao*)

These herbs were prepared and administered the same as above. In this formula, Ginseng, Atractylodes, Poria, and Glycyrrhiza (Licorice) strengthen the spleen. Pueraria gets rid of heat due to spleen deficiency. Agastaches eliminates dampness. And Auklandia helps to regulate the qi, thus helping to eliminate gas. I also counseled the mother on sticking to a clear, bland diet. Incidentally, the mother had a long history of chronic candidiasis which had eventually developed into multiple sclerosis. After four days, this child's mother reported that she still had lots of gas but that her thrush was getting better. "The white stuff was coming loose." I represcribed the same formula but added Radix Albus Paeoniae Lactiflorae (*Bai Shao*) to relieve the stomach cramps due to gas. After another two days, again the mother reported the thrush was still getting better.

161

There was still some gas but it did not seem to be so painful. We continued with this same formula for a total of 17 days after which there was no further thrush and no further colic.

9
How to Find a Chinese Medical Practitioner

Although Chinese medicine is more than 2,000 years old in Asia, Chinese medicine is in its infancy here in the West. In the United States, except for a few rare instances, Chinese medicine was confined to the Asian populations of various Chinatowns, Japan towns, and Korea towns in major, mainly costal cities. However, beginning in the mid-1970s, non-Asian Americans became interested in acupuncture. This coincided with President Nixon's historic trip to the People's Republic of China which "opened up" China to the Western world for the first time since the late 1940s.

Since acupuncture was the part of Chinese medicine which captured the public's attention, largely through news broadcasts on TV showing surgical operations performed with acupuncture anesthesia, the first schools of Chinese medicine to open in the West for the training of Western practitioners were self-styled acupuncture schools. By the early 1980s, states like California had created the first legislation allowing for the non-MD practice of acupuncture as a distinct and independent health care profession. At this point in time, more than half the states in the United States have legalized the independent practice of acupuncture by non-MDs. However, also early in the 1980s, teachers and students at these Western acupuncture colleges began to realize that there was a lot more to Chinese medicine than just acupuncture. Practitioners expressed more and more interest especially in Chinese herbal medicine, and now most Western schools of "acupuncture" also teach courses in Chinese herbal medicine.

Therefore, if one wants to find a professional practitioner of Chinese medicine in the West to take their children for treatment, they should look for someone who primarily advertises him/herself as an acupuncturist. In the United States, that means looking in the *Yellow Pages* under acupuncturists. However, there is great diversity in training and experience among Western acupuncturists. This means checking out the credentials of any potential practitioner. Below is a check-list of questions one should ask any potential acupuncturist you might be thinking of taking your child to see for treatment:

1. If acupuncture is legal in the state in which one lives, is the acupuncturist legally registered or licensed in that state? If not, why not? (It better be a real good reason.)
2. Is the practitioner a Diplomate of Acupuncture certified by the National Commission for the Certification of Acupuncturists (NCCA)?
3. If you are seeking help with Chinese herbal medicine, is the practitioner a Diplomate of Chinese Herbology certified by the NCCA?
4. Where did they get their training? How long was that training?
5. How long have they been in practice?
6. Have they been trained in TCM pediatrics?
7. Have they treated your child's disease or complaint before in other children and with what results?

Because many acupuncturists in the West are Asians who are not native English-speakers, be sure that you can communicate easily and effectively with the practitioner. The TCM practitioner is not just supposed to provide remedial treatment. He or she should be a source of guidance and instruction in how to live a healthier life. So be sure you can communicate with them. Otherwise you will only be getting a fraction of what Chinese medicine has to offer.

Remember that word of mouth referral from satisfied patients is one of the best possible recommendations for any practitioner. So do not be afraid to ask for the names and phone numbers of satisfied parents of children the practitioner has successfully treated. Because of practitioner/patient confidentiality, the practitioner will probably have to call you back with those names, since they are supposed to get permission first. In addition, health food store clerks often hear from their many customers who are the good practitioners in their community and they are often good people to ask for local referrals.

Below is the address and phone number of the National Commission for the Certification of Acupuncturists (NCCA). This is the commission which gives certification examinations for acupuncture and Chinese herbal medicine in the United States. You can call them for the names and addresses of diplomates near you. However, they cannot tell you who is good, bad, or better.

National Commission for the Certification of Acupuncturists (NCCA)
PO Box 97075 Washington, DC 20090-7075
Tel: 202-232-1404 Fax: 202-462-6157

Likewise, if acupuncture is legal in your state, you can call your State Department of Regulatory Agencies or the State Department of Health. They can then steer you to the right department for the names and addresses of local practitioners. It is sometimes possible to find out more about the credentials and expertise of individual practitioners by calling your state acupuncture professional association. Typically, whatever is the state agency which administers acupuncture in your state has the name and phone number of such state professional associations. Professional members of such associations must usually meet certain minimum levels of education and competence and adhere to a code of ethics.

Just as you would not call an electrician if you needed your plumbing fixed, I recommend prospective patients seek treatment only from fully qualified, professional practitioners of acupuncture and Chinese medicine. In order to sit for the NCCA exam, practitioners must have had not less than 1250 hours of specifically acupuncture education, and most American colleges of acupuncture and Oriental medicine require between 1800 and 2200 hours to graduate. Therefore, I strongly advise seeking out NCCA Diplomates of Acupuncture and Diplomates of Chinese Herbology.

10
Developmental Mileposts

Although not strictly a part of traditional Chinese pediatrics, many parents, and especially those who do not have a Western medical pediatrician, ask me if their child's development is normal. Below are some general guidelines for parents.

Height

Linear growth is measured with the child lying down on their back if the child is under 2 years of age. If the child is over 2, then they are measured standing up. Typically, infants height increases by 30% by 5 months and by more than 50% by 1 year old. After that, height doubles by 5 years of age. From then to puberty, growth slows down, and then at puberty speeds back up again.

Weight

Growth in weight roughly parallels that of growth in height. The infant doubles their weight by 5 months and triples it by their first birthday. They then quadruple their weight by 2 years old. Between 2 and 5 years of age, the annual increments of weight are fairly similar. After 5 years, weight gain slows down until puberty when it increases again along with the height.

Teething

As the reader most likely already knows, the baby's first set of teeth are not their permanent teeth. These baby teeth are shed like leaves and are, therefore, called deciduous teeth similar to deciduous leaves shed in the fall. In terms of when these baby or deciduous teeth come in, the lower incisors should come in somewhere between 5-9 months. From 8-12 months, the upper central incisors come in. From 10-12 months, the upper lateral incisors break through, and from 12-15 months the lower lateral incisors come out. The first molars come in between 10-16 months, the canines come in between 16 and 20 months, and the second molars break through somewhere between 20-30 months. These deciduous teeth are smaller than the permanent teeth which will replace them.

The second or permanent teeth begin to erupt somewhere after 5 years of age. For instance, the first molars come in between 5-7 years, the incisors erupt between 6-8 years, and the bicuspids break through between 9-12 years. Then the canines come in between 10-13 years, the second molars between 11-13 years, and the third molars between 17-25 years. These third molars are what are also called the wisdom teeth. Although both boys and girls develop their baby teeth at the same times, girls tend to get their permanent teeth earlier than boys.

Major developmental events

These are only rough guidelines. Individual children will do some of these things a bit earlier or later than others. When learning a new skill, it is common for the child to try something over and over without success, eventually becoming frustrated. Then they will not try that activity or skill for awhile. A bit later, they will suddenly be able to do that activity or skill as if from nowhere. Thus, often children will look like their development is going backwards when they are on the verge of making a new leap forward.

Birth

Newborns sleep most of the time. They can eat, clear their airway, and respond with crying to pain and displeasure.

Six weeks

By this time the child can look at objects in their line of sight. They can usually smile when spoken to and they can lie flat on their stomachs. If pulled into a sitting position, they cannot hold up their head, however.

Three months

By three months the child can smile spontaneously. They are vocalizing and they can follow a moving object with their eyes. They are capable of holding up their head themselves when sitting up and they can grasp objects placed in their hands.

Six months

By six months most children will be able to sit with support and to roll over. They can support themselves in a standing position, transfer objects from one hand to the other, and babble to toys.

Nine months

At nine months the child sits well, crawls, and pulls itself to a standing position. They usually say dada or mama, play pat-a-cake, and wave goodbye. They can also hold their own bottle.

One year

Most children this age can walk if held by their hand. They can speak several words and they can help to dress themselves.

Eighteen months

At this age the child walks well, can climb stairs holding on, turns several book pages at a time, speaks about 10 words, pulls toys on a string, and partially feeds itself.

Two years

By now most children run well, climb up and down stairs by themselves, turn single pages of a book at a time, can put on simple clothing, make simple 2-3 word sentences, and verbalize toilet needs. At this age, children are learning to be more independent, and necessarily so. Therefore, they often say no. For this reason, the age from 2-3 years is often called "the terrible twos."

Three years

The child can ride a tricycle, dresses well except for buttons and laces, counts to 10, uses plurals, questions constantly, and feeds itself well.

Four years

The child now alternates feet going up and down stairs, can throw a ball overhand, and can hop on one foot. They can copy a cross, they know at least one color, and can wash their hands and face. They also take care of their own toilet needs.

Five years

At this age, children can skip, catch a bounced ball, copy a triangle, know four colors, and dress and undress without assistance.

11
Resources for Going Further

For more information on Chinese medicine in general, see:

The Web That Has No Weaver: Understanding Chinese Medicine by Ted Kaptchuk, Congdon & Weed, NY, 1983. This is the best overall introduction to Chinese medicine for the serious lay reader. It has been a standard since it was first published over a dozen years ago and it has yet to be replaced.

Fundamentals of Chinese Medicine by the East Asian Medical Studies Society, Paradigm Publications, Brookline, MA, 1985. This is a more technical introduction and overview of TCM.

Traditional Medicine in Contemporary China by Nathan Sivin, Center for Chinese Studies, University of Michigan, Ann Arbor, 1987. This book discusses the development of Chinese medicine in China in the last half century.

Imperial Secrets of Health and Longevity by Bob Flaws, Blue Poppy Press, Inc., Boulder, CO, 1994. This book includes a section on Chinese dietary therapy and generally introduces the basic concepts of good health according to Chinese medicine.

Chinese Herbal Remedies by Albert Y. Leung, Universe Books, NY, 1984. This book is about simple Chinese herbal home remedies.

Legendary Chinese Healing Herbs by Henry C. Lu, Sterling Publishing, Inc., NY, 1991. This book is a fun way to begin learning about Chinese herbal medicine. It is full of interesting and entertaining anecdotes about Chinese medicinal herbs.

The Mystery of Longevity by Liu Zheng-cai, Foreign Languages Press, Beijing, 1990. This book is also about general principles and practice promoting good health according to Chinese medicine.

The National Alliance of Acupuncture & Oriental Medicine, 14637 Starr Rd, SE
Olalla, WA 98357
Tel. 206-851-6895 (or 6)
This is a national professional association which may be able to help with referrals.

The National Accreditation Commission for Schools & Colleges of Acupuncture & Oriental Medicine
1010 Wayne Ave., Suite 1270
Silver Springs, MD 20910
Tel. 301-608-9680
Fax: 301-608-9576
This national accreditation commission can provide information about accredited schools of acupuncture and Oriental medicine in the U.S.

For more information on Chinese dietary therapy, see:

Arisal of the Clear: A Simple Guide to Healthy Eating According to Traditional Chinese Medicine by Bob Flaws, Blue Poppy Press, Inc., Boulder, CO, 1991. This book is a layperson's primer on Chinese dietary therapy. It includes detailed sections on the clear, bland diet as well as sections on chronic candidiasis and allergies.

Prince Wen Hui's Cook: Chinese Dietary Therapy by Bob Flaws & Honora Lee Wolfe, Paradigm Publications, Brookline, MA, 1983. This book is an introduction to Chinese dietary therapy. Although some of the information it contains is dated, it does give the Chinese medicinal descriptions of most foods commonly eaten in the West.

The Book of Jook: Chinese Medicinal Porridges, A Healthy Alternative to the Typical Western Breakfast by Bob Flaws, Blue Poppy Press, Inc., Boulder, CO, 1995. This book is specifically about Chinese medicinal porridges made with very simple combinations of Chinese medicinal herbs.

The Tao of Nutrition by Maoshing Ni, Union of Tao and Man, Los Angeles, 1989

Harmony Rules: The Chinese Way of Health Through Food by Gary Butt & Frena Bloomfield, Samuel Weiser, Inc., York Beach, ME, 1985

Chinese System of Food Cures: Prevention & Remedies by Henry C. Lu, Sterling Publishing Co., Inc, NY, 1986

A Practical English-Chinese Library of Traditional Chinese Medicine: Chinese Medicated Diet ed. by Zhang En-qin, Shanghai College of Traditional Chinese Medicine Publishing House, Shanghai, 1990

Eating Your Way to Health — Dietotherapy in Traditional Chinese Medicine by Cai Jing-feng, Foreign Languages Press, Beijing, 1988

For more information on Chinese pediatric massage, see:

Chinese Pediatric Massage Therapy: A Parent's & Practitioner's Guide of the Treatment and Prevention of Childhood Disease by Fan Ya-li, Blue Poppy Press, Inc., Boulder, CO, 1994

A Parent's Guide to Chinese Pediatric Massage by Kyle Cline, Institute for Traditional Medicine, Portland, OR, 1993

Chinese Pediatric Massage, Practitioner's Reference Manual by Kyle Cline, Institute for Traditional Medicine, Portland, OR, 1993

Introduction to Chinese Pediatric Massage by Kyle Cline, Dharma Productions #302, Institute for Traditional Medicine, Portland, OR. This is a videotape

Chinese Pediatric Massage by Kyle Cline, Dharma Productions #301, Institute for Traditional Medicine, Portland, OR. This is also a videotape

Chinese Pediatric Massage: Parent's Reference Video by Kyle Cline, Dharma Productions #303, Institute for Traditional Medicine, Portland, OR. This, too, is a videotape

Infantile Tuina Therapy by Luan Chang-ye, Foreign Languages Press, Beijing, 1989

For more information on the relationship of chronic candidiasis, allergies, and autoimmune diseases, see:

Allergies and Candida by Steven Roschlitz, Human Ecology Balancing Sciences, 1991

Candida: The Symptoms, the Causes, the Cure by Luc de Schepper, self-published, Santa Monica, CA, 1990

Healthy at Last: Solutions to Chronic Ill Health by Cynthia Clinkscales, CEOM Publishing, Homer, AS, 1990

How to Prevent Yeast Infections, Yeast Consulting Services, P.O. Box 11157, Torrance, CA 90510

Solving the Puzzle of Your Hard-to-Raise Child by William G. Crook & Laura Stevens, Random House, NY, 1987

The Candida Albicans Yeast-free Cookbook by Pat Connolly, Keats Publishing, New Canaan, CT, 1985

The Candida Control Cookbook by Gail Burton, Aslan Publishing, Lower Lake, CA, 1993

The Yeast Connection, A Medical Breakthrough by William G. Crook, Vintage Books, NY, 1986. Although this book was first written in 1986, it is still the standard for lay readers on chronic candidiasis in English.

The Yeast Connection Cookbook, William G. Crook & Marjorie Hunt Jones, Professional Books, 1989

The Yeast Connection & Women by William G. Crook, Professional Books, 1995. Although the title says this book is for women, in fact, it contains all the up-dated materials Dr. Crook has learned about candidiasis since writing the above-mentioned book in the 1980's.

The Yeast Syndrome by John Parks Trowbridge & Martin Walker, Bantam Books, NY, 1988

For more information on possible side effects of immunizations, see:

DPT: A Shot in the Dark by Harris L. Coulter & Barbara Joe Fisher, Avery Publishing Group, NY

Immunization: The Reality Behind the Myth by Walene James, Bergin & Garvey, MA

Immunization: The Terrible Risks Your Children Face That Your Doctor Won't Reveal by Robert S. Mendelsohn, Second Opinion, 1993

Medicine: What Works & What Doesn't by the Editors of *What Doctors Don't Tell You*, Wallace Press, 1995

Vaccination and Immunization: Danger, Delusion and Alternatives by Leon Chaitow, C.W. Daniel Company Ltd.

For more information on antibiotics, see:

Beyond Antibiotics by Michael Schmidt, Lenden H. Smith & Keith W. Sehnert, North Atlantic Books, 1993

How to Raise A Healthy Child, In Spite of Your Doctor by Robert S. Mendelsohn, Contemporary Books, 1984

The Antibiotic Paradox: How Miracle Drugs are Destroying the Miracle by Stuart B. Levy, Plenum Press, 1992

The Plague Makers: How We Are Creating Catastrophe by Jeffrey Fisher, Simon & Schuster, NY, 1994

For mail order sources of Chinese medicinal herbs:

In the United States of America:

Spring Wind Herb Co.
2315 Fourth St.
Berkeley, CA 94710
Tel. 510-849-1820
Fax: 510-849-4886
Orders: 800-588-4883

China Herb Co.
165 W. Queen Lane
Philadelphia, PA 19144
Tel. 215-843-5864
Fax: 215-849-3338
Orders: 800-221-4372

Nuherbs Co.
3820 Penniman Ave.
Oakland, CA 94619
Tel. 415-534-4372
Orders: 800-233-4307

In the United Kingdom:

Acumedic Ltd.
101-105 Camden High St.
London NW1 7JN
Tel. 071-388-6704
Fax: 071-387-5766

East West Herb Shop
3 Neals Yard
Covent Garden, London WC2H 9DP
Tel. 071-379-1312
Fax: 071-379-4414

East West Herbs Ltd.
Langston Priory Mews
Kingham, Oxfordshire OX7 6UP
Tel. 01608-658862
Fax: 01608-658816

Harmony Acupuncture Supplies Center
629 High Road Leytonstone
London E11 4PA
Tel. 081-518-7337
Fax: 071-518-7338

Mayway Herbal Emporium
40 Sapcote Trading Estate, Dudden Hill
Lane
London NW10 2DJ
Tel. 081-459-1812
Fax: 081-459-1727

In Europe:

Homeofar n.v.
Hugo Verriestlaan
8500 Kortrijk, Belgium

China's Nature N.V.
Huyslaan 37
B-8790 Waregem
Tel: 32 (0)56 603307
Fax: 32 (0)56 612907

Tai Yang Chinese Herb Store
Elverdingsestrasse 90A
8900 Ieper, Belgium
Tel. 057-21-86-69
Fax: 057-21-97-78

Apotheek Gouka
Goenelaan 111
3114 CE Schiedam, Netherlands
Tel. 010-426-46-33
Fax: 010-473-08-45

Sinecura
Jurastrasse 23
5000 Aarau, Switzerland
Tel. 41-64-22-50-24
Fax: 41-64-22-52-69

P.P.C. Ltd.
Ireland
Tel. 091-753-222
Fax: 091-753-471

Dragon Herbs
Denmark
Tel. 44-66-21-14
Fax: 44-66-21-15

Euroherbs
Claassenland 15
NL-6932 AZ
Westervoort
Tel. O8-303-15660
Fax: 08-303-17752

Chinese Medical Center
Geldersekade 67-73
1011 EK Amsterdam
Tel. 31 020-623-50-60
Fax: 31 020-623-36-36

East West Herbs
Italy
Tel. 06-90-66-813
Fax: 06-90-66-813

East West Herbs
Spain
Tel. 1-539-0862
Fax: 1-639-0862

East West Herbs
Portugal
Tel. 1-486-4356
Fax: 1-486-4556

Harmonia I Naturalesa
L'Artisan Herboriste
BP 117
Andorra La Vella
ANDORA, via France
Tel: 33-376-835-566

In Australia:

Chianherb
29A Albion St.
Surry Hills, NSW 2010
Tel. 02-281-2122

Bibliography

Chinese language bibliography:

Er Ke Bing Liang Fang (Fine Formulas for Pediatric Diseases) by He Yuan-lin *et al.*, Yunnan University Press, Kunming, 1991

Er Ke Zheng Zhi (Pediatric Patterns & Treatments) by Cao Xu, Shanxi Science & Technology Press, Xian, 1980

Er Ke Zheng Zhi Xin Fa (The Heart Methods of Patterns & Treatments in Pediatrics) by Cheng Shao-en *et al.*, Beijing Science & Technology Press, Beijing, 1990

Jian Ming Xiao Er Tui Na (Simple, Clear Pediatric Tuina) by Zhang Shi-da *et al.*, Shanxi People's Press, Xian, 1983

Xiao Er Bing Zheng Wai Zhi Fa (External Treatment Methods in Pediatric Diseases & Conditions) by Zhang Qi-wen, Shandong Science & Technology Press, Jinan, 1991

Xiao Er Tui Na (Pediatric Tuina) by Jin Yi-cheng, Shanghai Science & Technology Press, Shanghai, 1981

Xiao Er Xiao Hua Bu Liang (Pediatric Indigestion) by Zhou Run-zhi *et al.*, People's Health & Hygiene Press, Beijing, 1985

You Ke Tie Jing (The Iron Mirror of Pediatrics) by Xia Jiang, Qing dynasty, Chinese National Press, Beijing, 1987

You You Ji Cheng (Comprehensive Pediatrics) by Chen Fu-zheng, Yuan dynasty, People's Army Press, Beijing, 1988

Zhi You Xin Shu (The Heart Book of Treating Children) by Ceng Shi-rong, Yuan dynasty, Beijing Municipal Chinese National Book Store, Beijing, 1985

Zhong Yi Er Ke Lin Chuang Shou Ce (A Clinical Handbook of Chinese Medicine Pediatrics) by the Shanghai College of Traditional Chinese Medicine, Shanghai Science & Technology Press, Shanghai, 1983

Zhong Yi Er Ke Zheng Zhi (Chinese Medicine Pediatrics Patterns & Treatments) by Zhou Tian-xin, Guangdong Science & Technology Press, Guangzhou, 1990

Zhong Yi Er Ke Xue (A Study of Chinese Medicine Pediatrics) by the Guangdong College of Traditional Chinese Medicine, Shanghai Science & Technology Press, Shanghai, 1981

Zhong Yi Er Ke Xue (A Study of Chinese Medicine Pediatrics) by Guo Zhen-qiu, Shanghai Science & Technology Press, Shanghai, 1983

Zhong Yi Er Ke Xue (A Study of Chinese Medicine Pediatrics) by Jiang You-ren *et al.*, Shanghai Science & Technology Press, Shanghai, 1991

Zhong Yi Er Ke Xue (A Study of Chinese Medicine Pediatrics) by the Shanghai College of Traditional Chinese Medicine & the Shanghai Municipal Department of Health & Hygiene, People's Health & Hygiene Press, Beijing, 1983

Zhong Yi Zi Xue Cong Shu (Chinese Medicine Self-study Collection of Books): Er Ke (Pediatrics) by Yang Yi-ya, Hebei Science & Technology Press, Shijiazhuang, 1987

English language bibliography:

Acupuncture in the Treatment of Children, Revised Edition by Julian Scott, Eastland Press, Seattle, WA, 1992

A Barefoot Doctor's Manual, Revised & Enlarged Edition prepared by the Revolutionary Health Committee of Hunan Province, Cloudburst Press, Mayne Isle & Seattle, 1977

Essentials of Traditional Chinese Pediatrics by Cao Ji-ming *et al.*, Foreign Languages Press, Beijing, 1990

Pediatric Bronchitis: Its TCM Cause, Diagnosis, Treatment & Prevention by Xiao Shu-qin *et al.*, Blue Poppy Press, Inc., Boulder, CO, 1991

The English-Chinese Encyclopedia of Practical Traditional Chinese Medicine: Paediatrics ed. by Xu Xiang-cai, Higher Education Press, Beijing, 1991

The Merck Manual, 15th Edition ed. by Robert Berkow, Merck Sharp & Dohme Research Laboratories, Rahway, NJ, 1987

Index

OTHER BOOKS ON CHINESE MEDICINE
AVAILABLE FROM BLUE POPPY PRESS
3450 Penrose Place, Suite 110, Boulder, CO 80301
For ordering 1-800-487-9296 PH. 303\447-8372 FAX 303\245-8362

A NEW AMERICAN ACUPUNCTURE by Mark Seem, ISBN 0-936185-44-9

ACUPOINT POCKET REFERENCE ISBN 0-936185-93-7

ACUPUNCTURE AND MOXIBUSTION FORMULAS & TREATMENTS by Cheng Dan-an, trans. by Wu Ming, ISBN 0-936185-68-6

ACUTE ABDOMINAL SYNDROMES: Their Diagnosis & Treatment by Combined Chinese-Western Medicine by Alon Marcus, ISBN 0-936185-31-7

AGING & BLOOD STASIS: A New Approach to TCM Geriatrics by Yan De-xin, ISBN 0-936185-63-5

AIDS & ITS TREATMENT ACCORDING TO TRADITIONAL CHINESE MEDICINE by Huang Bing-shan, trans. by Fu-Di, ISBN 0-936185-28-7

BETTER BREAST HEALTH NATURALLY with CHINESE MEDICINE by Honora Lee Wolfe & Bob Flaws ISBN 0-936185-90-2

THE BOOK OF JOOK: Chinese Medicinal Porridges, An Alternative to the Typical Western Break-fast by B. Flaws, ISBN0-936185-60-0

CHINESE MEDICAL PALMISTRY: Your Health in Your Hand by Zong Xiao-fan & Gary Liscum, ISBN 0-936185-64-3

CHINESE MEDICINAL TEAS: Simple, Proven, Folk Formulas for Common Diseases & Promoting Health by Zong Xiao-fan & Gary Liscum, ISBN 0-936185-76-7

CHINESE MEDICINAL WINES & ELIXIRS by Bob Flaws, ISBN 0-936185-58-9

CHINESE PEDIATRIC MASSAGE THERAPY: *A Parent's & Practitioner's Guide to the Prevention & Treatment of Childhood Illness* by Fan Ya-li, ISBN 0-936185-54-6

CHINESE SELF-MASSAGE THERAPY: The Easy Way to Health by Fan Ya-li ISBN 0-936185-74-0

A COMPENDIUM OF TCM PATTERNS & TREATMENTS Bob Flaws & Dan Finney, ISBN 0-936185-70-8

CURING ARTHRITIS NATURALLY WITH CHINESE MEDICINE by Doug Frank & Bob Flaws ISBN 0-936185-87-2

CURING DEPRESSION NATURALLY WITH CHINESE MEDICINE by Rosa Schnyer & B. Flaws ISBN 0-936185-94-5

CURING HAY FEVER NATURALLY WITH CHINESE MEDICINE by Bob Flaws, ISBN 0-936185-91-0

CURING HEADACHES NATURALLY WITH CHINESE MEDICINE, Bob Flaws, ISBN 0-936185-95-3

CURING INSOMNIA NATURALLY WITH CHINESE MEDICINE by Bob Flaws ISBN 0-936185-85-6

CURING PMS NATURALLY WITH CHINESE MEDICINE by Bob Flaws ISBN 0-936185-85-6

THE DAO OF INCREASING
LONGEVITY AND CONSERVING
ONE'S LIFE by Anna Lin & Bob Flaws, ISBN
0-936185-24-4

THE DIVINE FARMER'S MATERIA
MEDICA (*A Translation of the Shen Nong Ben Cao*) by Yang Shou-zhong ISBN 0-936185-96-1

THE DIVINELY RESPONDING
CLASSIC: *A Translation of the Shen Ying Jing from Zhen Jiu Da Cheng*, trans. by Yang Shou-zhong & Liu Feng-ting ISBN 0-936185-55-4

DUI YAO: THE ART OF COMBINING
CHINESE HERBAL MEDICINALS by
Philippe Sionneau ISBN 0-936185-81-3

ENDOMETRIOSIS, INFERTILITY AND
TRADITIONAL CHINESE MEDICINE:
A Laywoman's Guide by Bob Flaws ISBN 0-936185-14-7

THE ESSENCE OF LIU FENG-WU'S
GYNECOLOGY by Liu Feng-wu, translated by
Yang Shou-zhong ISBN 0-936185-88-0

EXTRA TREATISES BASED ON INVES-
TIGATION & INQUIRY: *A Translation of
Zhu Dan-xi's Ge Zhi Yu Lun*, by Yang Shou-zhong
& Duan Wu-jin, ISBN 0-936185-53-8

FIRE IN THE VALLEY: TCM Diagnosis &
Treatment of Vaginal Diseases ISBN 0-936185-25-2

FU QING-ZHU'S GYNECOLOGY trans. by
Yang & Liu ISBN 0-936185-35-X

FULFILLING THE ESSENCE: A
*Handbook of Traditional & Contemporary
Treatments for Female Infertility* by Bob Flaws,
ISBN 0-936185-48-1

GOLDEN NEEDLE WANG LE-TING: A
20th Century Master's Approach to Acupuncture by Yu Hui-chan and Han Fu-ru, trans. by
Shuai Xue-zhong

A HANDBOOK OF TRADITIONAL
CHINESE DERMATOLOGY by Liang Jian-
hui, trans. Zhang & Flaws, ISBN 0-936185-07-4

A HANDBOOK OF TRADITIONAL
CHINESE GYNECOLOGY by Zhejiang
College of TCM, trans. by Zhang Ting-liang, ISBN
0-936185-06-6 (4th edit.)

A HANDBOOK OF MENSTRUAL DIS-
EASES IN CHINESE MEDICINE by Bob
Flaws ISBN 0-936185-82-1

A HANDBOOK of TCM PEDIATRICS by
Bob Flaws, ISBN 0-936185-72-4

A HANDBOOK OF TCM UROLOGY &
MALE SEXUAL DYSFUNCTION by Anna
Lin, OMD, ISBN 0-936185-36-8

THE HEART & ESSENCE OF DAN-XI'S
METHODS OF TREATMENT by Xu Dan-
xi, ISBN 0-926185-49-X

THE HEART TRANSMISSION OF
MEDICINE by Liu Yi-ren, trans. by Yang
Shou-zhong ISBN 0-936185-83-X

HIGHLIGHTS OF ANCIENT ACU-
PUNCTURE PRESCRIPTIONS. trans. by
Wolfe & Crescenz ISBN 0-936185-23-6

How to Have A HEALTHY PREGNANCY,
HEALTHY BIRTH with Chinese Medicine
by Honora Lee Wolfe, ISBN 0-936185-40-6

HOW TO WRITE A TCM HERBAL
FORMULA: *A Logical Methodology for the
Formulation & Administration of Chinese Herbal
Medicine in Decoction* by Flaws, ISBN 0-936185-49-X

IMPERIAL SECRETS OF HEALTH &
LONGEVITY by Flaws, ISBN 0-936185-51-1

KEEPING YOUR CHILD HEALTHY WITH CHINESE MEDICINE by Bob Flaws, ISBN 0-936185-71-6

THE LAKESIDE MASTER'S STUDY OF THE PULSE by Li Shi-zhen, trans. by Bob Flaws, ISBN 1-891845-01-2

Li Dong-yuan's TREATISE ON THE SPLEEN & STOMACH, *A Translation of the Pi Wei Lun* by Yang Shou-zhong & Li Jian-yong, ISBN 0-936185-41-4

LOW BACK PAIN: Care & Prevention with Chinese Medicine by Douglas Frank, ISBN 0-936185-66-X

MASTER HUA'S CLASSIC OF THE CENTRAL VISCERA by Hua Tuo, ISBN 0-936185-43-0

MASTER TONG'S ACUPUNCTURE: An Ancient Alternative Style in Modern Clinical Practice by M. Lee 0-926185-37-6

THE MEDICAL I CHING: *Oracle of the Healer Within* by Miki Shima, OMD, ISBN 0-936185-38-4

MANAGING MENOPAUSE NATURALLY with Chinese Medicine by Honora Wolfe ISBN 0-936185-98-8

PAO ZHI: Introduction to Processing Chinese Medicinals to Enhance Their Therapeutic Effect, by Philippe Sionneau, ISBN 0-936185-62-1

PATH OF PREGNANCY, Vol. I, Gestational Disorders by Flaws, ISBN 0-936185-39-2
PATH OF PREGNANCY, Vol. II, Postpartum Diseases by Flaws. ISBN 0-936185-42-2

PEDIATRIC BRONCHITIS: Its Cause, Diagnosis & Treatment According to TCM trans. Gao Yu-li ISBN 0-936185-26-0

PRINCE WEN HUI'S COOK: Chinese Dietary Therapy by Bob Flaws & Honora Lee Wolfe, ISBN 0-912111-05-4, $12.95 (Published by Paradigm Press)

THE PULSE CLASSIC: A Translation of the *Mai Jing* by Wang Shu-he, trans. by Yang Shou-zhong ISBN 0-936185-75-9

THE SECRET OF CHINESE PULSE DIAGNOSIS by Bob Flaws, ISBN 0-936185-67-8

SEVENTY ESSENTIAL TCM FORMULAS FOR BEGINNERS by Bob Flaws, ISBN 0-936185-59-7

SHAOLIN SECRET FORMULAS for Treatment of External Injuries, by De Chan, ISBN 0-936185-08-2

STATEMENTS OF FACT IN TRADITIONAL CHINESE MEDICINE by Bob Flaws, ISBN 0-936185-52-X

STICKING TO THE POINT 1: A Rational Methodology for the Step by Step Formulation & Administration of an Acupuncture Treatment by Bob Flaws ISBN 0-936185-17-1

STICKING TO THE POINT 2: A Study of Acupuncture & Moxibustion Formulas and Strategies by Bob Flaws ISBN 0-936185-97-X

A STUDY OF DAOIST ACUPUNCTURE & MOXIBUSTION by Liu Zheng-cai ISBN 1-891845-08-X

THE SYSTEMATIC CLASSIC OF ACUPUNCTURE & MOXIBUSTION (*Jia Yi Jing*) by Huang-fu Mi, trans. by Yang Shou-zhong & Charles Chace, ISBN 0-936185-29-5

TEACH YOURSELF TO READ MODERN MEDICAL CHINESE by Bob Flaws, ISBN 0-936185-99-6

THE TAO OF HEALTHY EATING ACCORDING TO CHINESE MEDICINE by Bob Flaws, ISBN 0-936185-92-9

THE TREATMENT OF DISEASE IN TCM, Vol I: Diseases of the Head & Face Including Mental/Emotional Disorders by Philippe Sionneau & Lü Gang, ISBN 0-936185-69-4

THE TREATMENT OF DISEASE IN TCM, Vol. II: Diseases of the Eyes, Ears, Nose, & Throat by Sionneau & Lü, ISBN 0-936185-69-4

THE TREATMENT OF DISEASE, Vol. III: Diseases of the Mouth, Lips, Tongue, Teeth & Gums, by Sionneau & Lü, ISBN 0-936185-79-1

THE TREATMENT OF DISEASE, Vol. IV: Diseases of the Neck, Shoulders, Back, & Limbs, by Sionneau & Lü, ISBN 0-936185-89-9

THE TREATMENT OF DISEASE, Vol. V: Diseases of the Chest & Abdomen, by Sionneau & Lü, ISBN 1-891845-02-0

THE TREATMENT OF EXTERNAL DISEASES WITH ACUPUNCTURE & MOXIBUSTION by Yan Cui-lan and Zhu Yun-long, ISBN 0-936185-80-5

260 ESSENTIAL CHINESE MEDICINALS by Bob Flaws, ISBN 1-891845-03-9

630 QUESTIONS & ANSWERS ABOUT CHINESE HERBAL MEDICINE: A WORKBOOK & STUDY GUIDE by Bob Flaws ISBN 1-891845-04-7

SIGIL

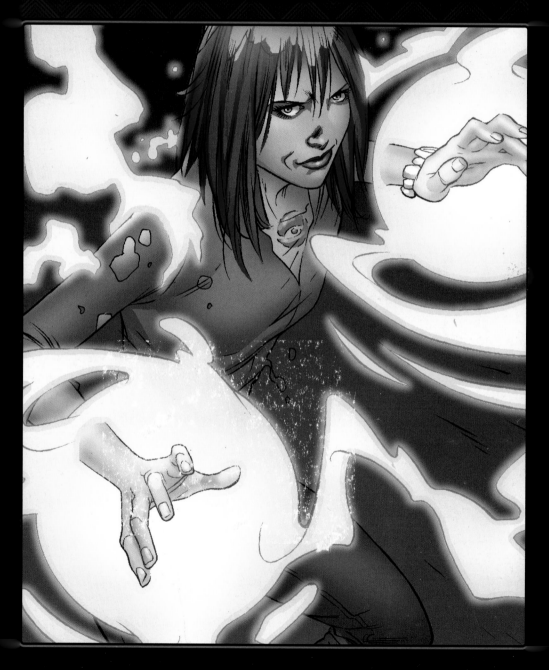

OUT OF TIME

SIGIL

OUT OF TIME

Writer
MIKE CAREY

Penciler
LEONARD KIRK
WITH **PAT OLLIFFE**
(#2, pages 16-19 & #3, pages 17-20)

Inker
ED TADEO
WITH **PAT DAVIDSON**
(#3, pages 14-20)

Colorist
GURU EFX

Letterer
ROB STEEN

Cover Art
JELENA DJURDJEVIC

Assistant Editors
SEBASTIAN GIRNER & JAKE THOMAS

Senior Editor
NICK LOWE

COLLECTION EDITOR: JENNIFER GRÜNWALD • EDITORIAL ASSISTANTS: JAMES EMMETT & JOE HOCHSTEIN
ASSISTANT EDITORS: ALEX STARBUCK & NELSON RIBEIRO • EDITOR, SPECIAL PROJECTS: MARK D. BEAZLEY
SENIOR EDITOR, SPECIAL PROJECTS: JEFF YOUNGQUIST • SENIOR VICE PRESIDENT OF SALES: DAVID GABRIEL
SENIOR VICE PRESIDENT OF BRAND PLANNING & COMMUNICATIONS: MICHAEL PASCIULLO
COVER DESIGN: PATRICK MCGRATH • SENIOR VICE PRESIDENT OF CREATIVE: TOM MARVELLI

EDITOR IN CHIEF: AXEL ALONSO • CHIEF CREATIVE OFFICER: JOE QUESADA
PUBLISHER: DAN BUCKLEY • EXECUTIVE PRODUCER: ALAN FINE

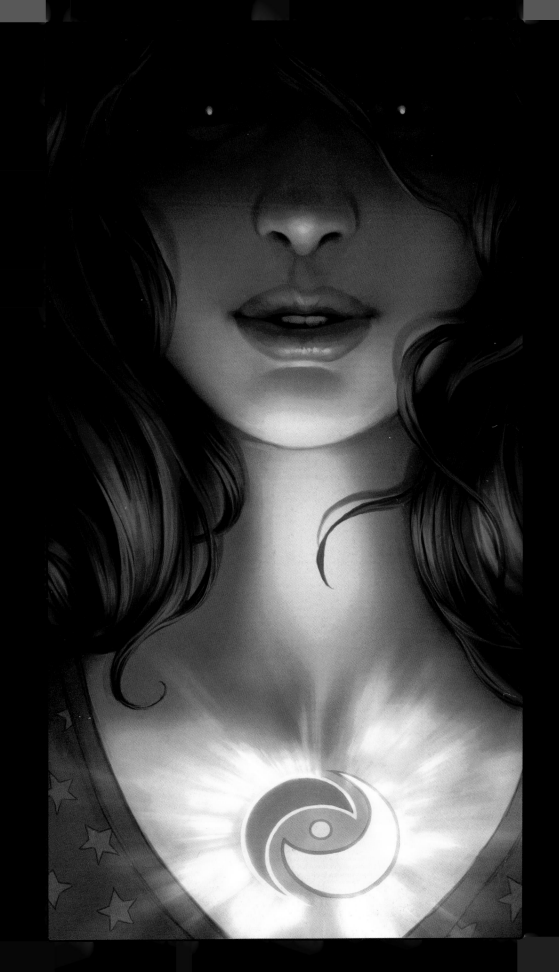

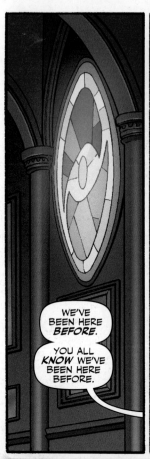

WE'VE BEEN HERE *BEFORE.*

YOU ALL *KNOW* WE'VE BEEN HERE BEFORE.

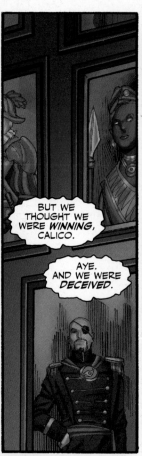

BUT WE THOUGHT WE WERE *WINNING,* CALICO.

AYE. AND WE WERE *DECEIVED.*

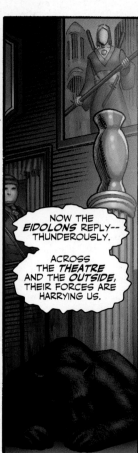

NOW THE *EIDOLONS* REPLY-- THUNDEROUSLY.

ACROSS THE *THEATRE* AND THE *OUTSIDE,* THEIR FORCES ARE HARRYING US.

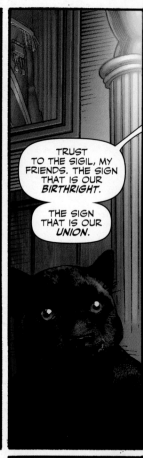

TRUST TO THE SIGIL, MY FRIENDS. THE SIGN THAT IS OUR *BIRTHRIGHT.*

THE SIGN THAT IS OUR *UNION.*

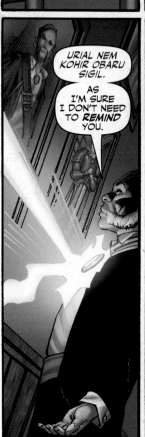

URIAL NEM KOHIR OBARU SIGIL.

AS I'M SURE I DON'T NEED TO *REMIND* YOU.

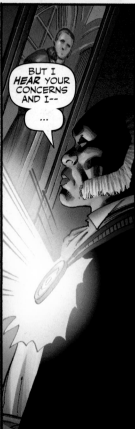

BUT I *HEAR* YOUR CONCERNS AND I--

...

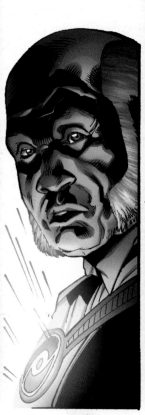

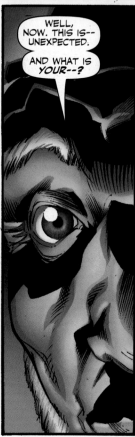

WELL, NOW. THIS IS-- UNEXPECTED.

AND WHAT IS *YOUR--?*

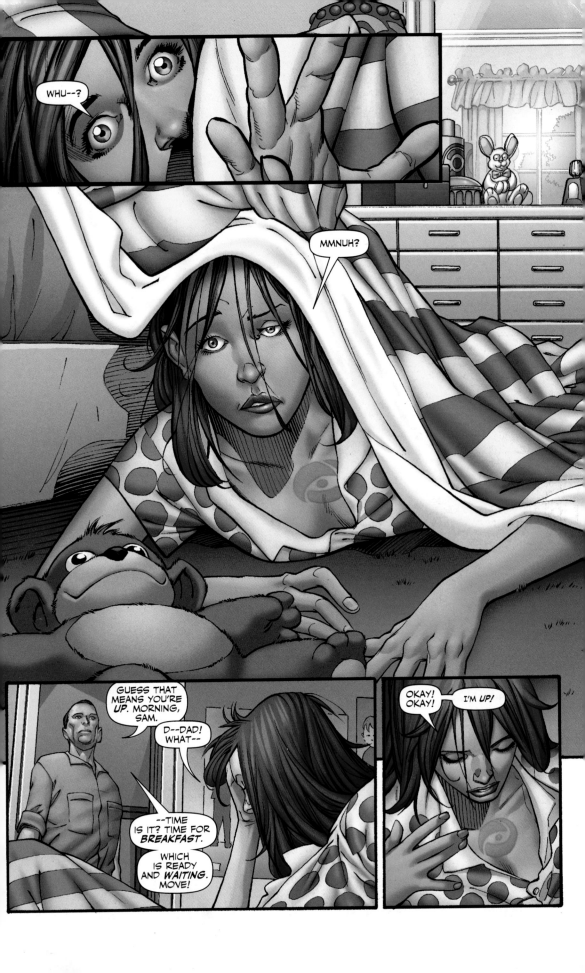

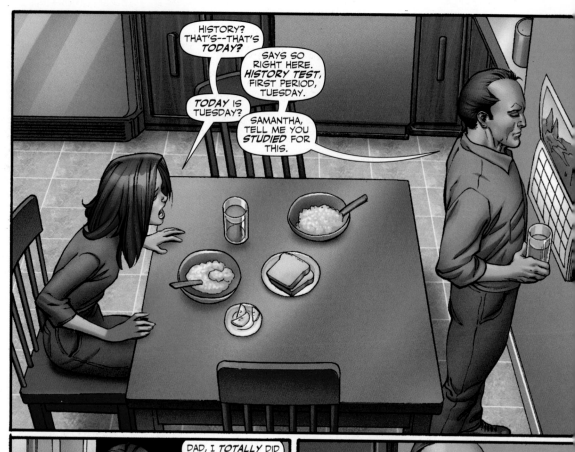

HISTORY? THAT'S--THAT'S *TODAY?*

SAYS SO RIGHT HERE. *HISTORY TEST,* FIRST PERIOD, TUESDAY.

TODAY IS TUESDAY?

SAMANTHA, TELL ME YOU *STUDIED* FOR THIS.

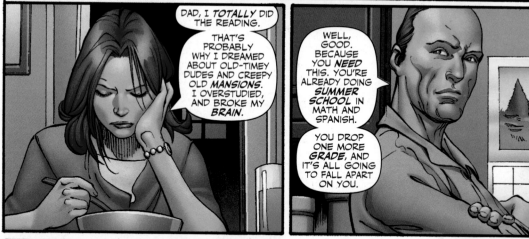

DAD, I *TOTALLY* DID THE READING.

THAT'S PROBABLY WHY I DREAMED ABOUT OLD-TIMEY DUDES AND CREEPY OLD *MANSIONS.* I OVERSTUDIED, AND BROKE MY *BRAIN.*

WELL, GOOD. BECAUSE YOU *NEED* THIS. YOU'RE ALREADY DOING *SUMMER SCHOOL* IN MATH AND SPANISH.

YOU DROP ONE MORE *GRADE,* AND IT'S ALL GOING TO FALL APART ON YOU.

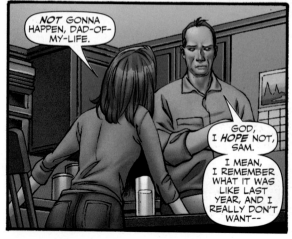

NOT GONNA HAPPEN, DAD-OF-MY-LIFE.

GOD, I *HOPE* NOT, SAM. I MEAN, I REMEMBER WHAT IT WAS LIKE LAST YEAR, AND I REALLY DON'T WANT--

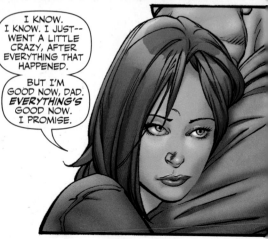

I KNOW. I KNOW. I JUST-- WENT A LITTLE CRAZY, AFTER EVERYTHING THAT HAPPENED.

BUT I'M GOOD NOW, DAD. *EVERYTHING'S* GOOD NOW. I PROMISE.

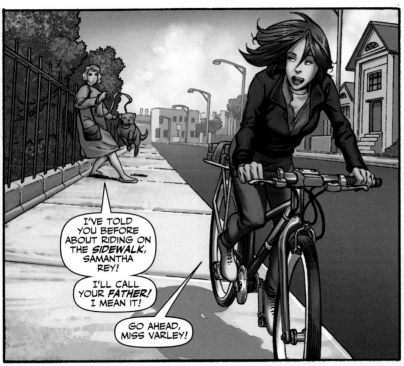

I'VE TOLD YOU BEFORE ABOUT RIDING ON THE *SIDEWALK,* SAMANTHA REY!

I'LL CALL YOUR *FATHER!* I MEAN IT!

GO AHEAD, MISS VARLEY!

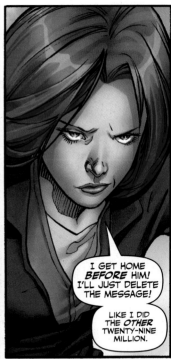

I GET HOME *BEFORE* HIM! I'LL JUST DELETE THE MESSAGE!

LIKE I DID THE *OTHER* TWENTY-NINE MILLION.

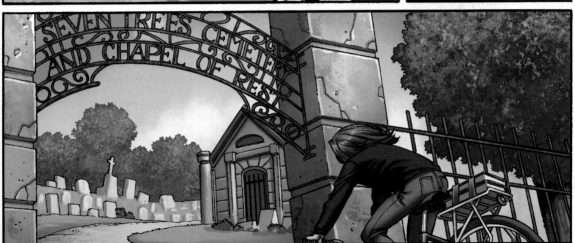

SEVEN TREES CEMETERY AND CHAPEL OF REST

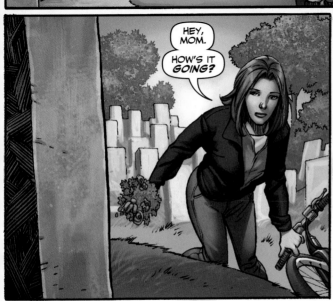

HEY, MOM.

HOW'S IT *GOING?*

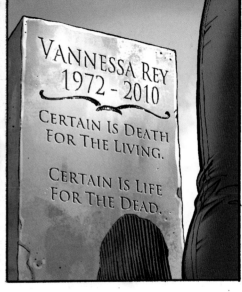

VANNESSA REY
1972 - 2010

CERTAIN IS DEATH FOR THE LIVING.

CERTAIN IS LIFE FOR THE DEAD.

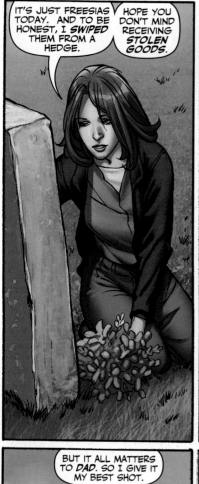

IT'S JUST FREESIAS TODAY. AND TO BE HONEST, I *SWIPED* THEM FROM A HEDGE.

HOPE YOU DON'T MIND RECEIVING *STOLEN GOODS*.

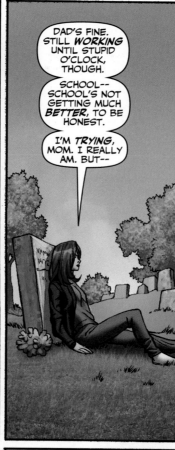

DAD'S FINE. STILL *WORKING* UNTIL STUPID O'CLOCK, THOUGH.

SCHOOL-- SCHOOL'S NOT GETTING MUCH *BETTER*, TO BE HONEST.

I'M *TRYING*, MOM. I REALLY AM. BUT--

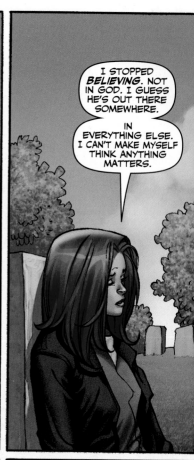

I STOPPED *BELIEVING*. NOT IN GOD. I GUESS HE'S OUT THERE SOMEWHERE.

IN EVERYTHING ELSE. I CAN'T MAKE MYSELF THINK ANYTHING MATTERS.

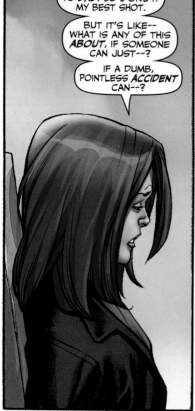

BUT IT ALL MATTERS TO *DAD*. SO I GIVE IT MY BEST SHOT.

BUT IT'S LIKE-- WHAT IS ANY OF THIS *ABOUT*, IF SOMEONE CAN JUST--?

IF A DUMB, POINTLESS *ACCIDENT* CAN--?

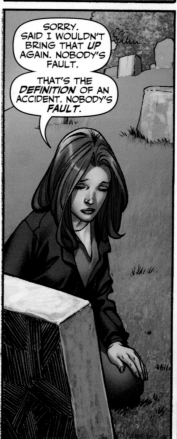

SORRY. SAID I WOULDN'T BRING THAT *UP* AGAIN. NOBODY'S FAULT.

THAT'S THE *DEFINITION* OF AN ACCIDENT. NOBODY'S *FAULT*.

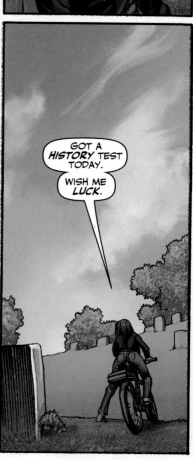

GOT A *HISTORY* TEST TODAY.

WISH ME *LUCK*.

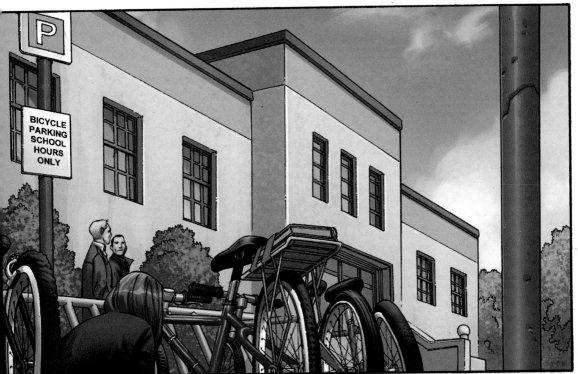

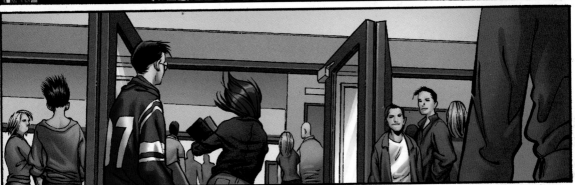

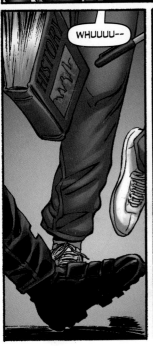

WHUUUU--

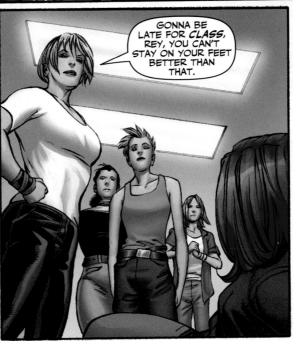

GONNA BE LATE FOR *CLASS*, REY, YOU CAN'T STAY ON YOUR FEET BETTER THAN THAT.

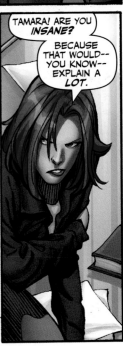

TAMARA! ARE YOU *INSANE?*

BECAUSE THAT WOULD-- YOU KNOW-- EXPLAIN A *LOT.*

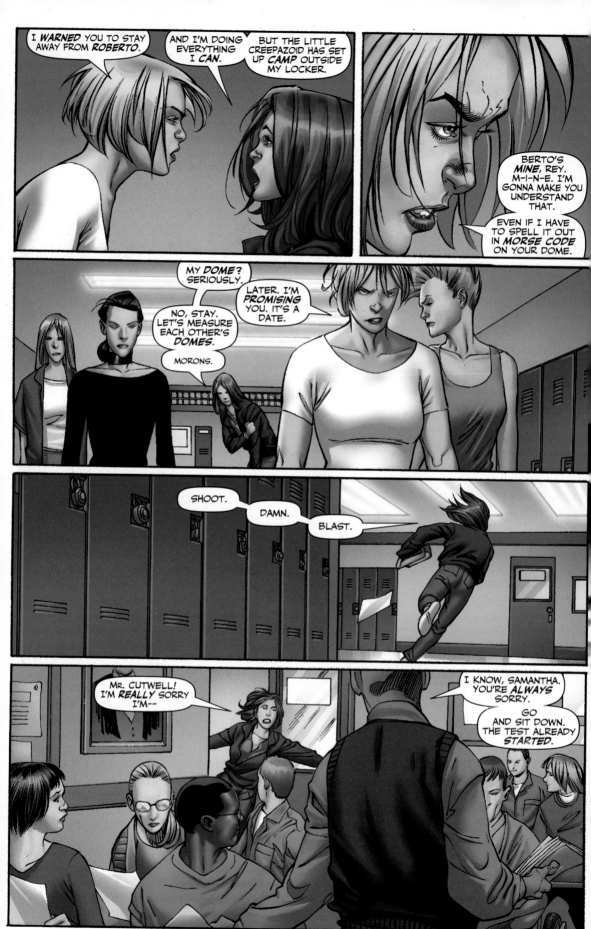

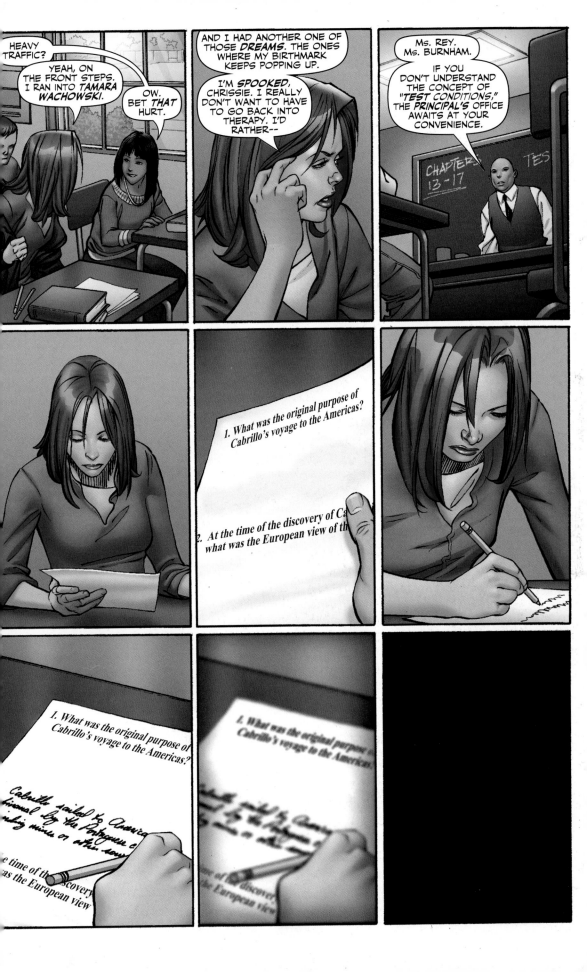

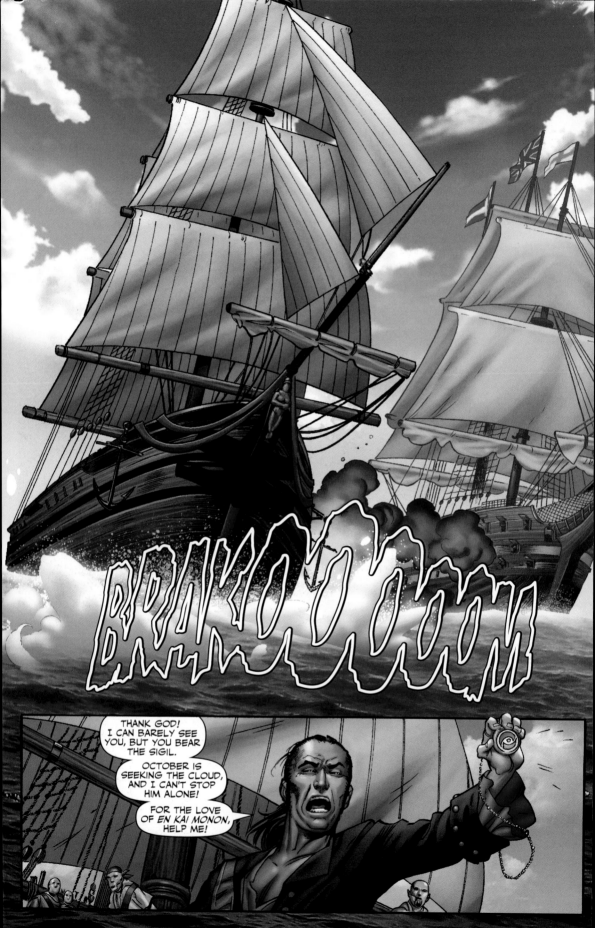

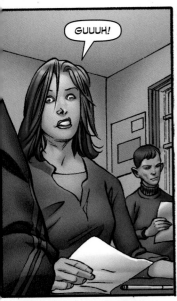

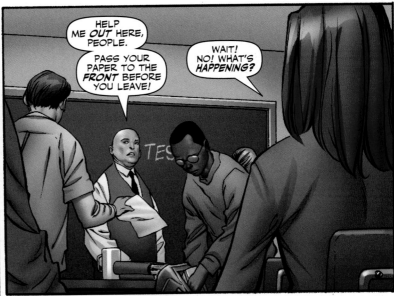

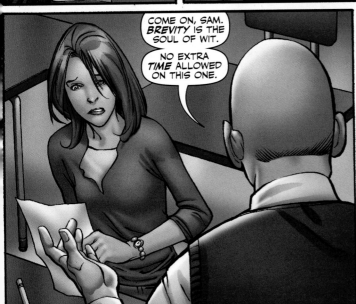

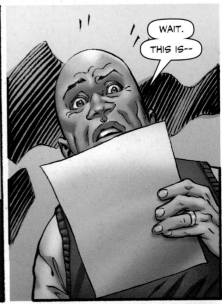

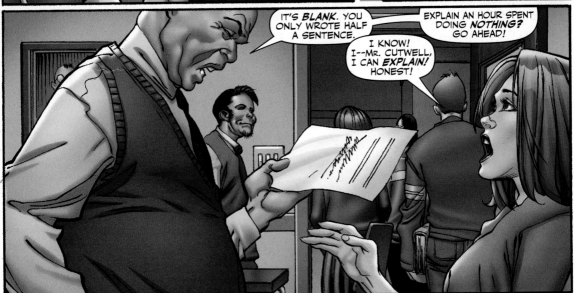

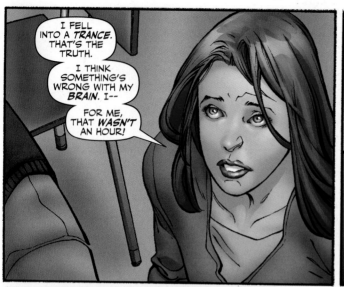

I FELL INTO A *TRANCE.* THAT'S THE TRUTH.

I THINK SOMETHING'S WRONG WITH MY *BRAIN.* I--

FOR ME, THAT *WASN'T* AN HOUR!

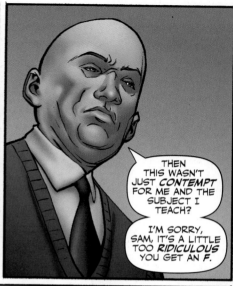

THEN THIS WASN'T JUST *CONTEMPT* FOR ME AND THE SUBJECT I TEACH?

I'M SORRY, SAM, IT'S A LITTLE TOO *RIDICULOUS* YOU GET AN *F.*

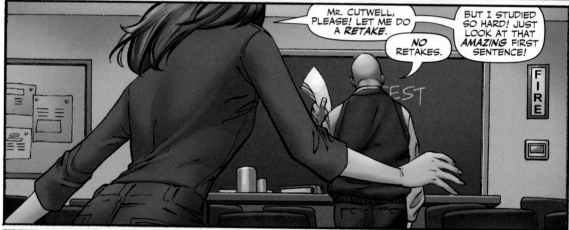

MR. CUTWELL, PLEASE! LET ME DO A *RETAKE.*

NO RETAKES.

BUT I STUDIED SO HARD! JUST LOOK AT THAT *AMAZING* FIRST SENTENCE!

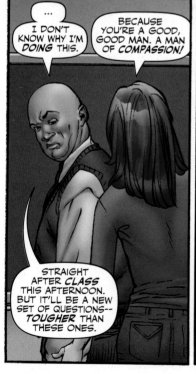

...

I DON'T KNOW WHY I'M *DOING* THIS.

BECAUSE YOU'RE A GOOD, GOOD MAN. A MAN OF *COMPASSION!*

STRAIGHT AFTER *CLASS* THIS AFTERNOON. BUT IT'LL BE A NEW SET OF QUESTIONS-- *TOUGHER* THAN THESE ONES.

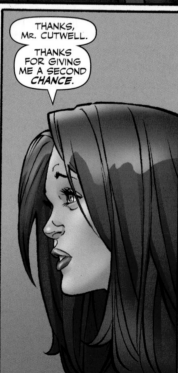

THANKS, MR. CUTWELL.

THANKS FOR GIVING ME A SECOND *CHANCE.*

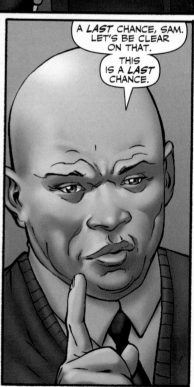

A *LAST* CHANCE, SAM. LET'S BE CLEAR ON THAT.

THIS IS A *LAST* CHANCE.

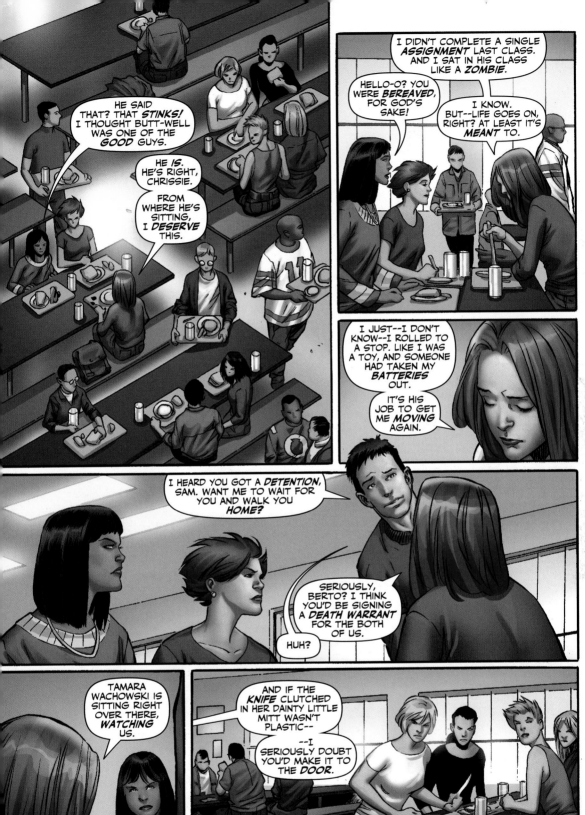

HE SAID THAT? THAT *STINKS!* I THOUGHT BUTT-WELL WAS ONE OF THE *GOOD* GUYS.

HE *IS.* HE'S RIGHT, CHRISSIE.

FROM WHERE HE'S SITTING, I *DESERVE* THIS.

I DIDN'T COMPLETE A SINGLE *ASSIGNMENT* LAST CLASS. AND I SAT IN HIS CLASS LIKE A *ZOMBIE.*

HELLO-O? YOU WERE *BEREAVED,* FOR GOD'S SAKE!

I KNOW. BUT--LIFE GOES ON, RIGHT? AT LEAST IT'S *MEANT* TO.

I JUST--I DON'T KNOW--I ROLLED TO A STOP. LIKE I WAS A TOY, AND SOMEONE HAD TAKEN MY *BATTERIES* OUT.

IT'S HIS JOB TO GET ME *MOVING* AGAIN.

I HEARD YOU GOT A *DETENTION,* SAM. WANT ME TO WAIT FOR YOU AND WALK YOU *HOME?*

SERIOUSLY, BERTO? I THINK YOU'D BE SIGNING A *DEATH WARRANT* FOR THE BOTH OF US.

HUH?

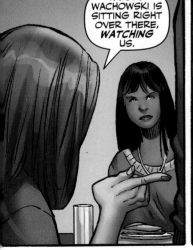

TAMARA WACHOWSKI IS SITTING RIGHT OVER THERE, *WATCHING* US.

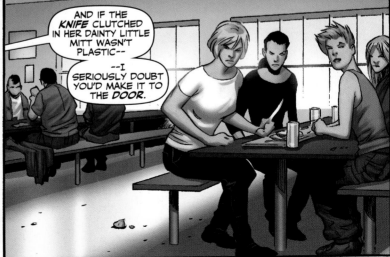

AND IF THE *KNIFE* CLUTCHED IN HER DAINTY LITTLE MITT WASN'T PLASTIC--

--I SERIOUSLY DOUBT YOU'D MAKE IT TO THE *DOOR.*

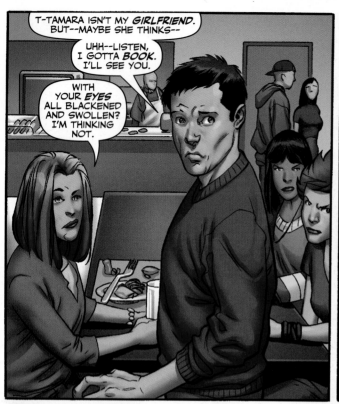

T-TAMARA ISN'T MY *GIRLFRIEND*. BUT--MAYBE SHE THINKS--

UHH--LISTEN, I GOTTA *BOOK*. I'LL SEE YOU.

WITH YOUR *EYES* ALL BLACKENED AND SWOLLEN? I'M THINKING *NOT*.

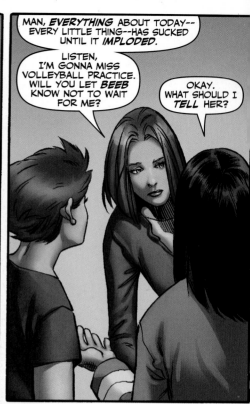

MAN, *EVERYTHING* ABOUT TODAY-- EVERY LITTLE THING--HAS SUCKED UNTIL IT *IMPLODED*.

LISTEN, I'M GONNA MISS VOLLEYBALL PRACTICE. WILL YOU LET *BEEB* KNOW NOT TO WAIT FOR ME?

OKAY. WHAT SHOULD I *TELL* HER?

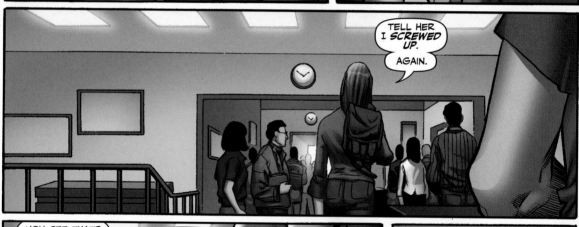

TELL HER I *SCREWED* UP.

AGAIN.

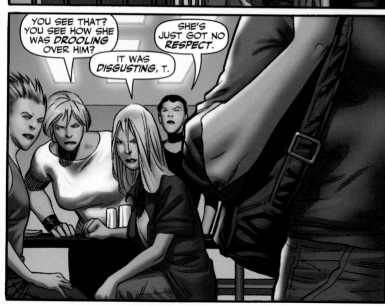

YOU SEE THAT? YOU SEE HOW SHE WAS *DROOLING* OVER HIM?

SHE'S JUST GOT NO *RESPECT*.

IT WAS *DISGUSTING*, T.

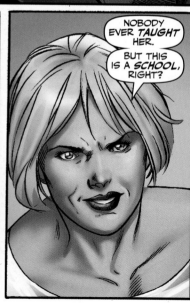

NOBODY EVER *TAUGHT* HER.

BUT THIS IS A *SCHOOL*, RIGHT?

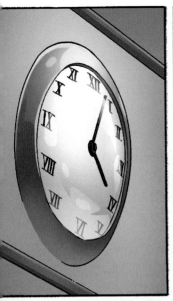

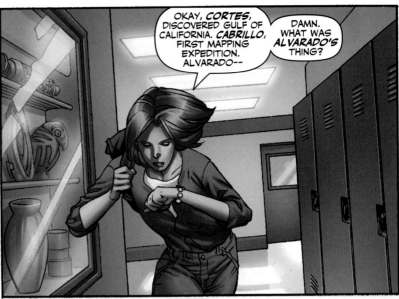

OKAY, *CORTES*, DISCOVERED GULF OF CALIFORNIA. *CABRILLO*, FIRST MAPPING EXPEDITION. ALVARADO--

DAMN. WHAT WAS *ALVARADO'S* THING?

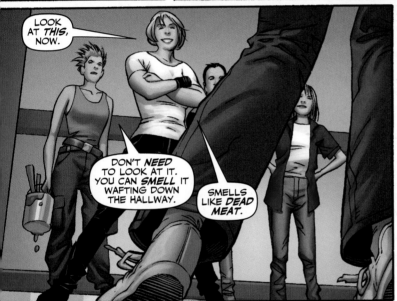

LOOK AT *THIS*, NOW.

DON'T *NEED* TO LOOK AT IT. YOU CAN *SMELL* IT WAFTING DOWN THE HALLWAY.

SMELLS LIKE *DEAD MEAT*.

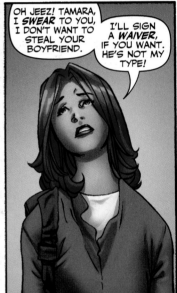

OH JEEZ! TAMARA, I *SWEAR* TO YOU, I DON'T WANT TO STEAL YOUR BOYFRIEND.

I'LL SIGN A *WAIVER*, IF YOU WANT. HE'S NOT MY TYPE!

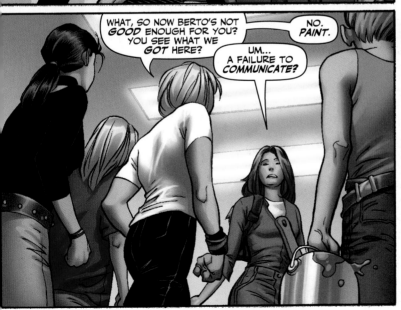

WHAT, SO NOW BERTO'S NOT *GOOD* ENOUGH FOR YOU? YOU SEE WHAT WE *GOT* HERE?

UM... A FAILURE TO *COMMUNICATE?*

NO. *PAINT*.

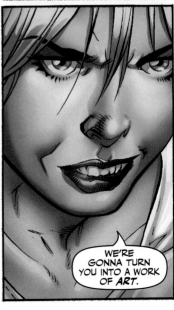

WE'RE GONNA TURN YOU INTO A WORK OF *ART*.

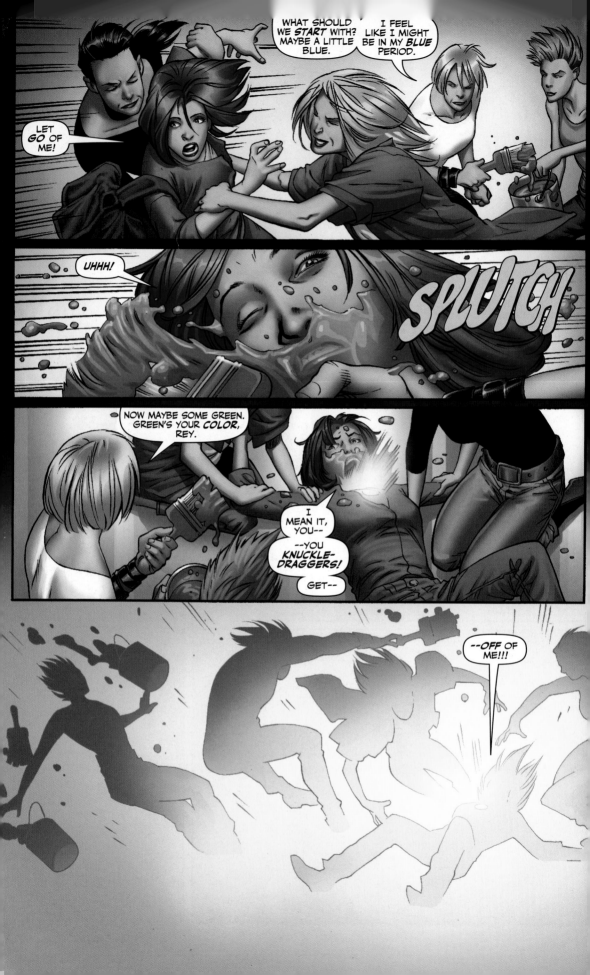

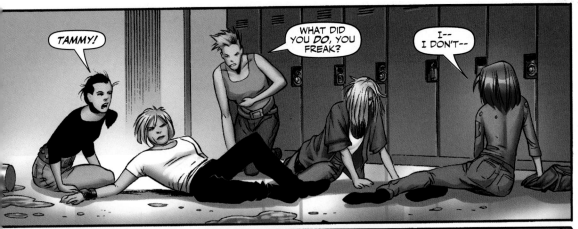

TAMMY!

WHAT DID YOU *DO*, YOU FREAK?

I-- I DON'T--

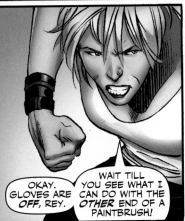

OKAY. GLOVES ARE *OFF*, REY.

WAIT TILL YOU SEE WHAT I CAN DO WITH THE *OTHER* END OF A PAINTBRUSH!

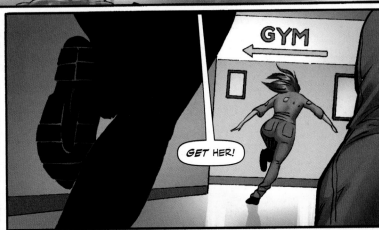

GYM

GET HER!

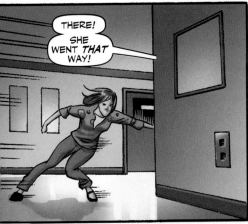

THERE! SHE WENT *THAT* WAY!

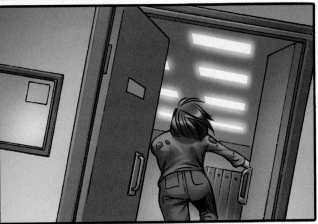

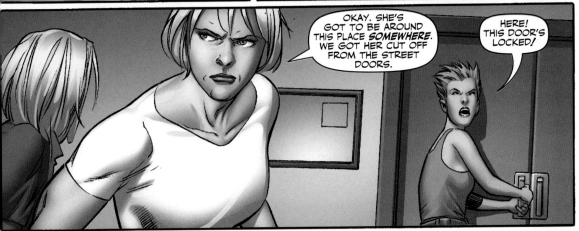

OKAY. SHE'S GOT TO BE AROUND THIS PLACE *SOMEWHERE*. WE GOT HER CUT OFF FROM THE STREET DOORS.

HERE! THIS DOOR'S LOCKED!

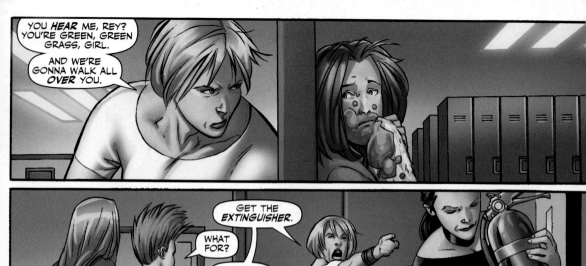

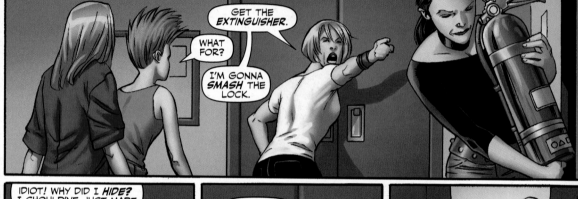

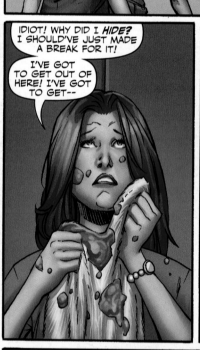

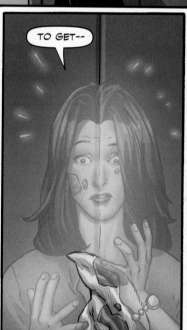

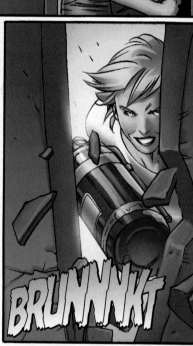

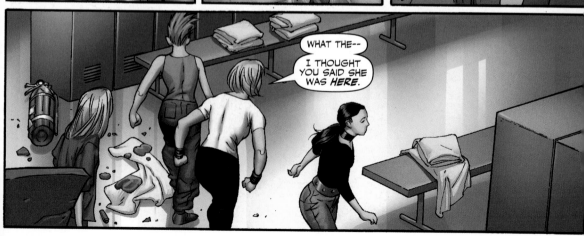

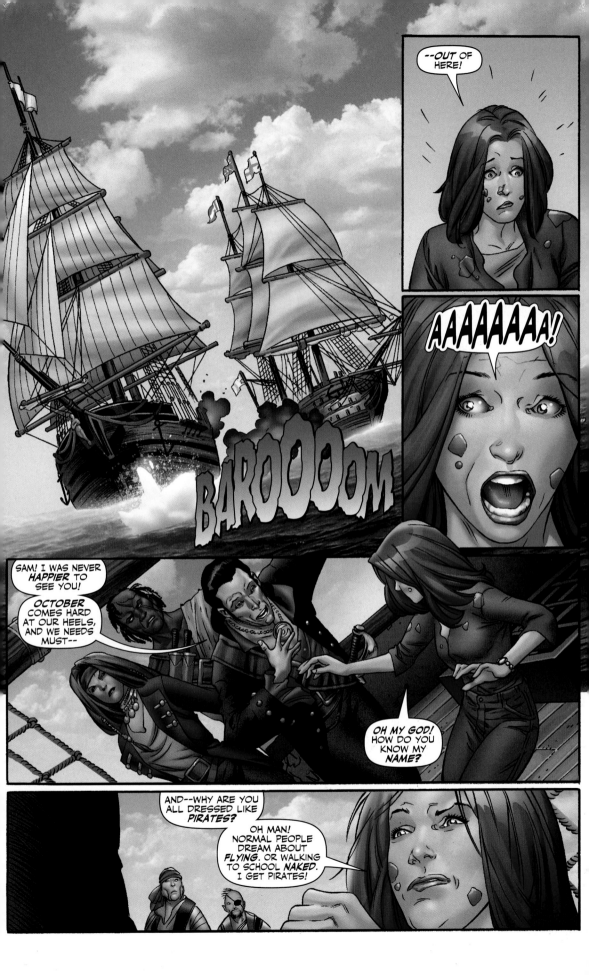

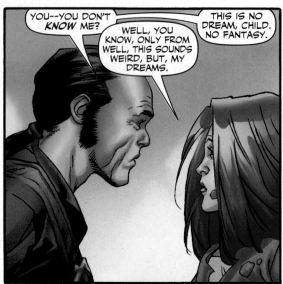

YOU--YOU DON'T *KNOW* ME?

WELL, YOU KNOW, ONLY FROM WELL, THIS SOUNDS WEIRD, BUT, MY DREAMS.

THIS IS NO DREAM, CHILD. NO FANTASY.

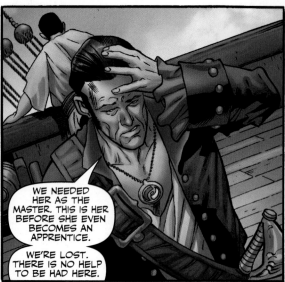

WE NEEDED HER AS THE MASTER. THIS IS HER BEFORE SHE EVEN BECOMES AN APPRENTICE.

WE'RE LOST. THERE IS NO HELP TO BE HAD HERE.

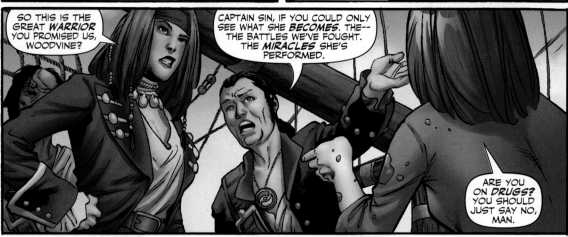

SO THIS IS THE GREAT *WARRIOR* YOU PROMISED US, WOODVINE?

CAPTAIN SIN, IF YOU COULD ONLY SEE WHAT SHE *BECOMES*. THE-- THE BATTLES WE'VE FOUGHT. THE *MIRACLES* SHE'S PERFORMED.

ARE YOU ON *DRUGS?* YOU SHOULD JUST SAY NO, MAN.

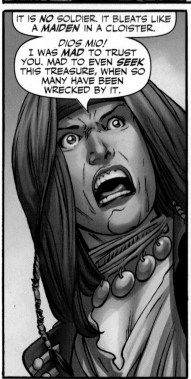

IT IS *NO* SOLDIER. IT BLEATS LIKE A *MAIDEN* IN A CLOISTER.

DIOS MIO! I WAS *MAD* TO TRUST YOU. MAD TO EVEN *SEEK* THIS TREASURE, WHEN SO MANY HAVE BEEN WRECKED BY IT.

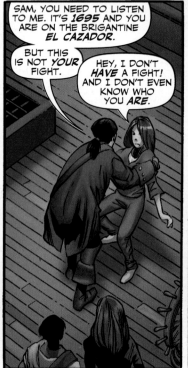

SAM, YOU NEED TO LISTEN TO ME. IT'S *1695* AND YOU ARE ON THE BRIGANTINE *EL CAZADOR*.

BUT THIS IS NOT *YOUR* FIGHT.

HEY, I DON'T *HAVE* A FIGHT! AND I DON'T EVEN KNOW WHO YOU *ARE*.

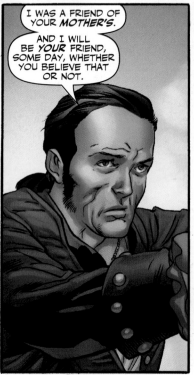

I WAS A FRIEND OF YOUR *MOTHER'S*.

AND I WILL BE *YOUR* FRIEND, SOME DAY, WHETHER YOU BELIEVE THAT OR NOT.

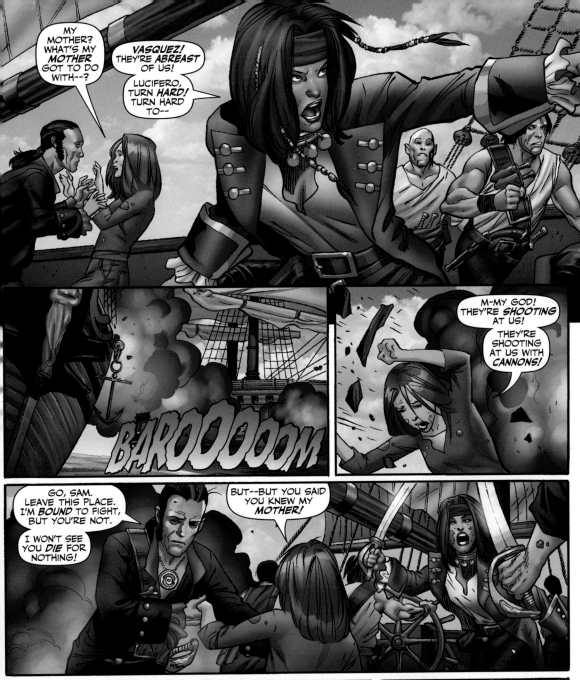

MY MOTHER? WHAT'S MY MOTHER GOT TO DO WITH--?

VASQUEZ! THEY'RE ABREAST OF US!

LUCIFERO, TURN HARD! TURN HARD TO--

M-MY GOD! THEY'RE SHOOTING AT US!

THEY'RE SHOOTING AT US WITH CANNONS!

BAROOOOOM

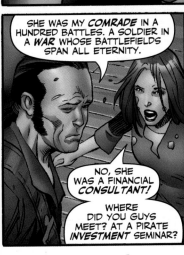

GO, SAM. LEAVE THIS PLACE. I'M BOUND TO FIGHT, BUT YOU'RE NOT.

I WON'T SEE YOU DIE FOR NOTHING!

BUT--BUT YOU SAID YOU KNEW MY MOTHER!

SHE WAS MY COMRADE IN A HUNDRED BATTLES. A SOLDIER IN A WAR WHOSE BATTLEFIELDS SPAN ALL ETERNITY.

NO, SHE WAS A FINANCIAL CONSULTANT!

WHERE DID YOU GUYS MEET? AT A PIRATE INVESTMENT SEMINAR?

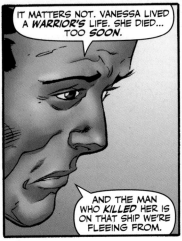

IT MATTERS NOT. VANESSA LIVED A WARRIOR'S LIFE. SHE DIED... TOO SOON.

AND THE MAN WHO KILLED HER IS ON THAT SHIP WE'RE FLEEING FROM.

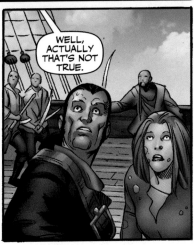

WELL, ACTUALLY THAT'S NOT TRUE.

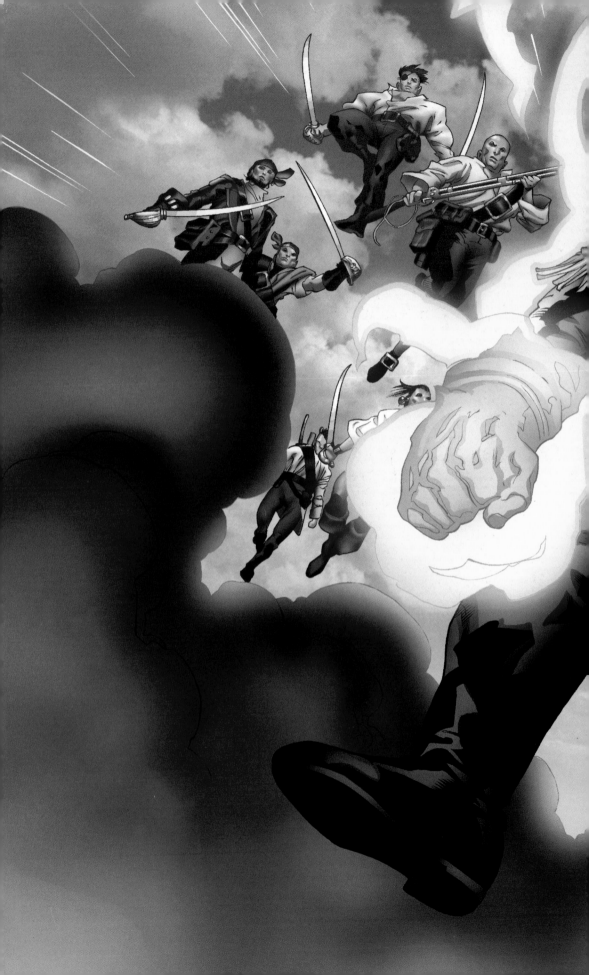

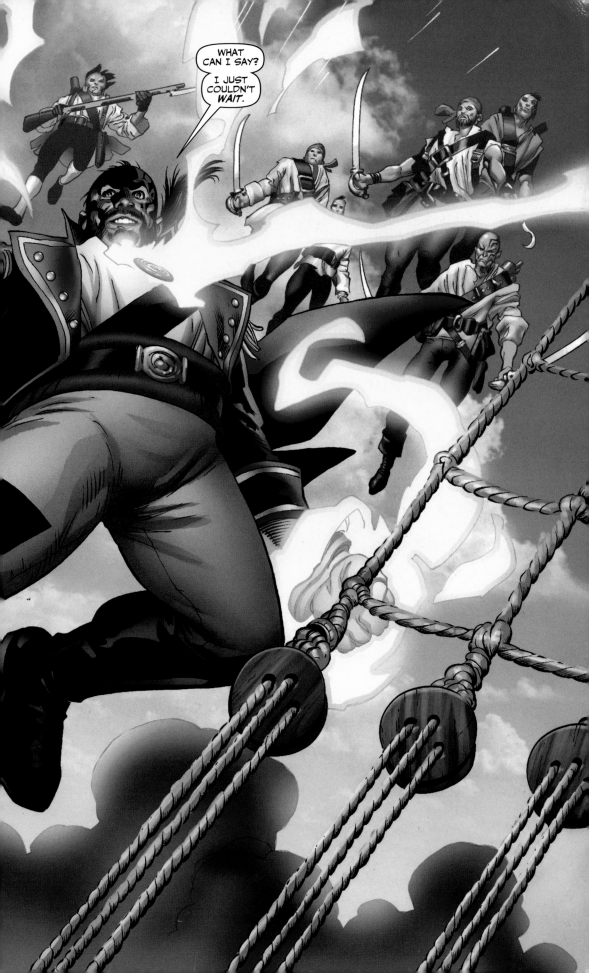

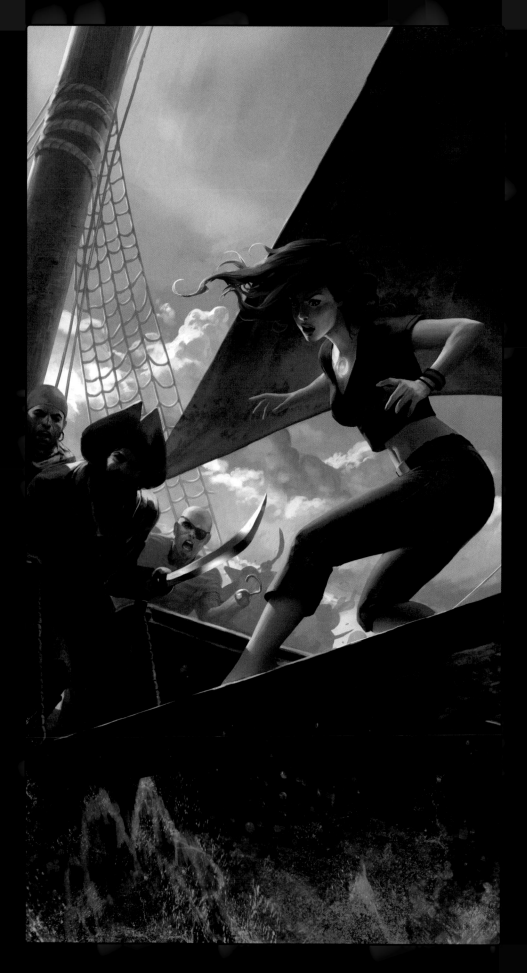

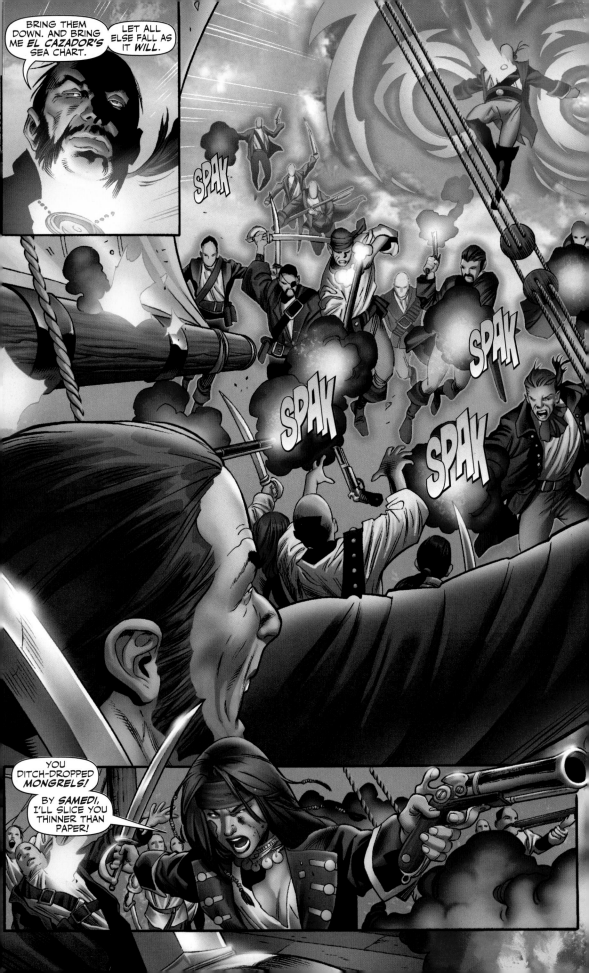

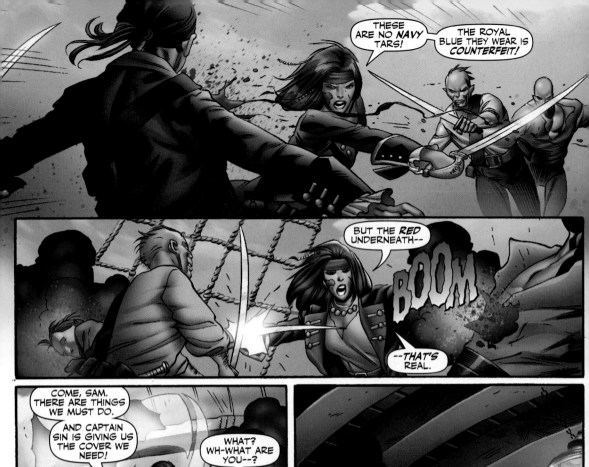

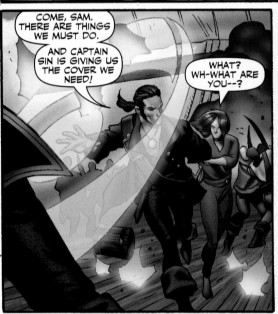

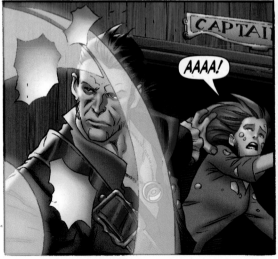

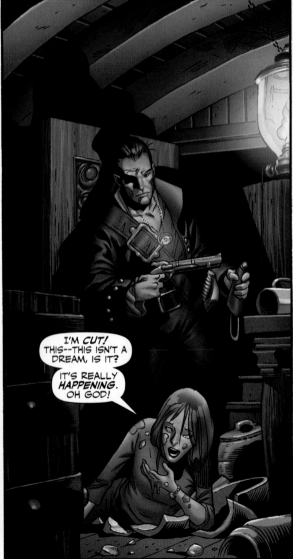

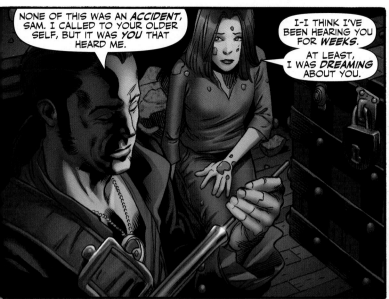

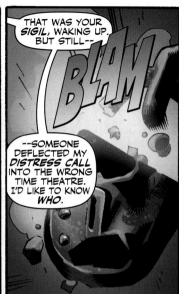

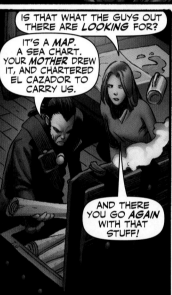

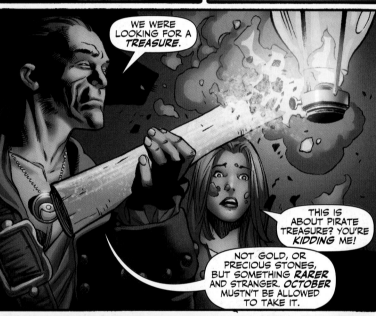

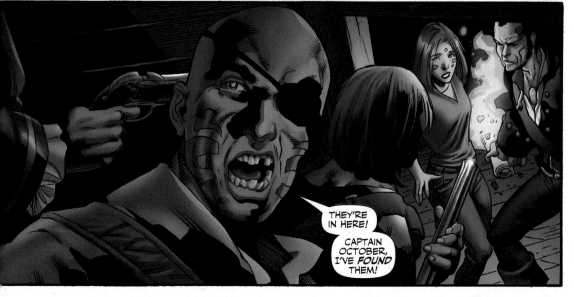

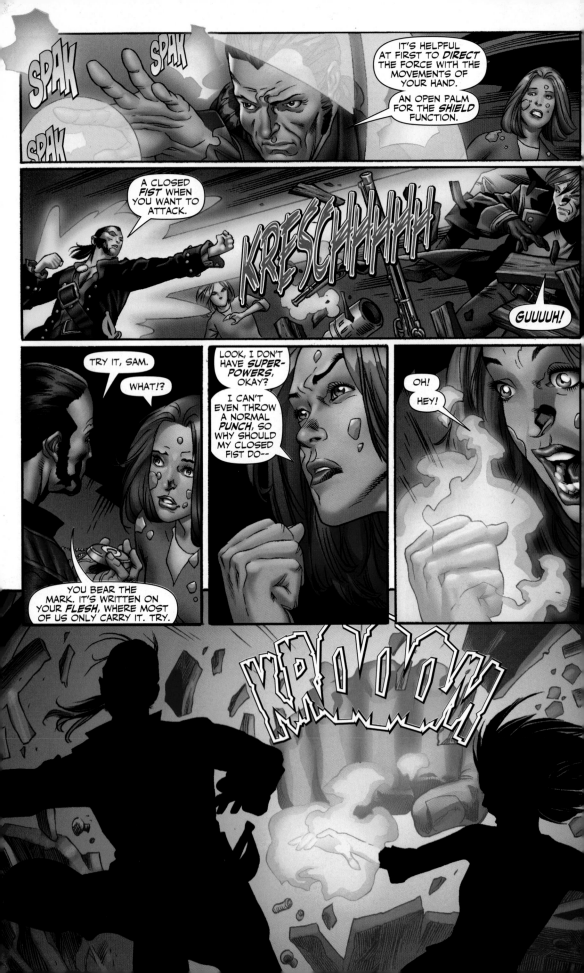

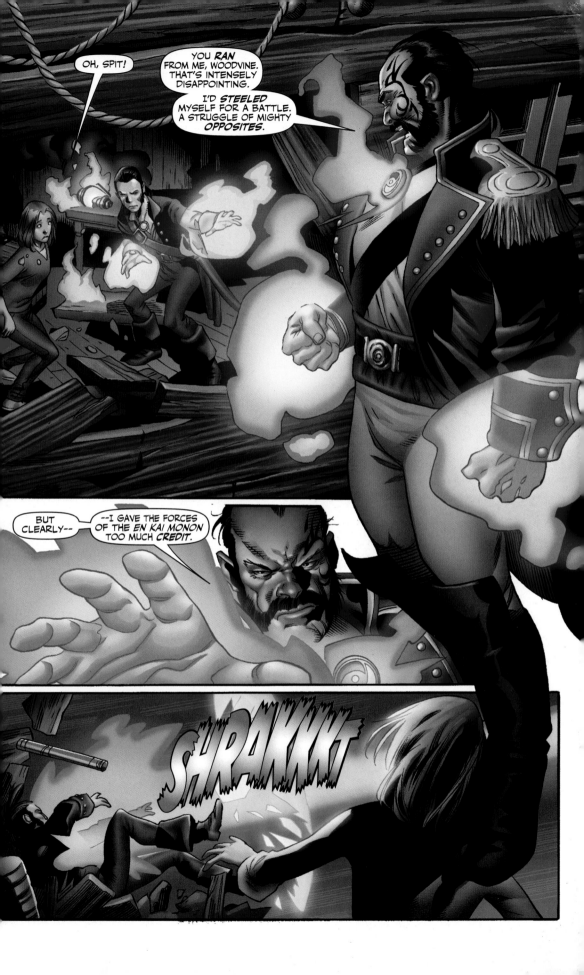

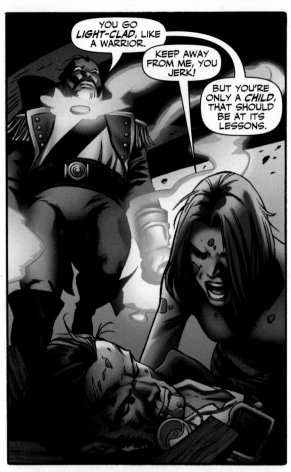
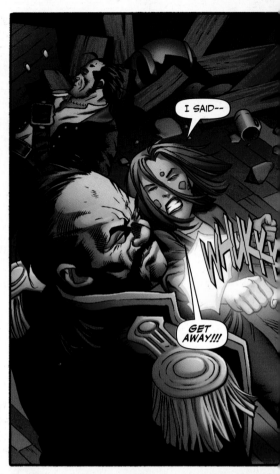
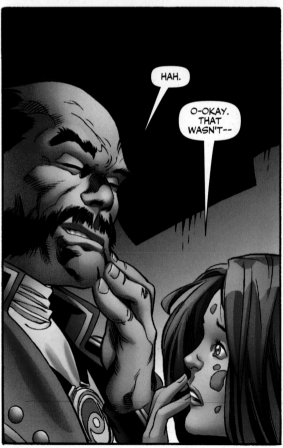
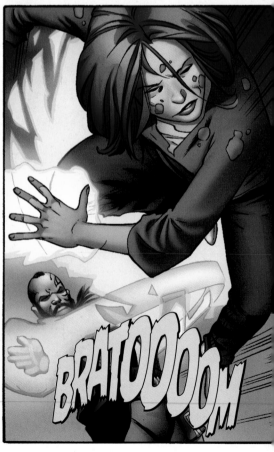

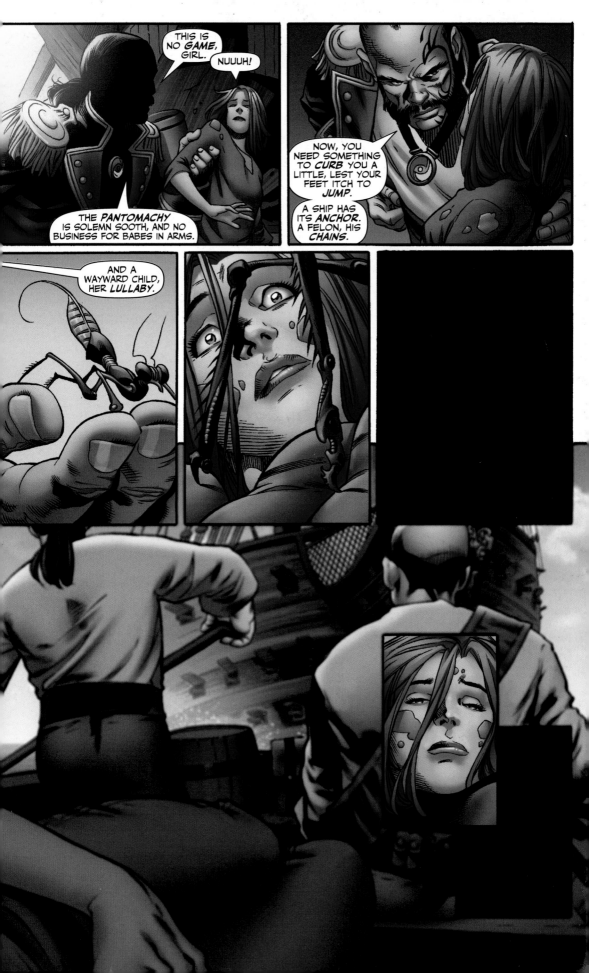

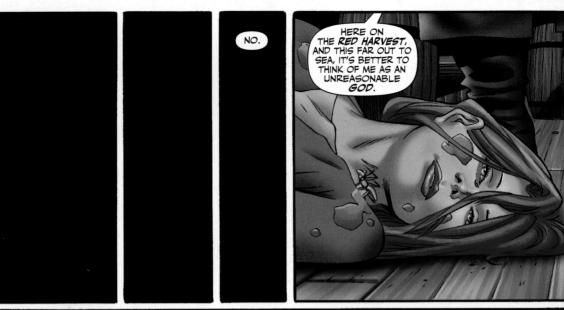

NO.

HERE ON THE *RED HARVEST*, AND THIS FAR OUT TO SEA, IT'S BETTER TO THINK OF ME AS AN UNREASONABLE *GOD*.

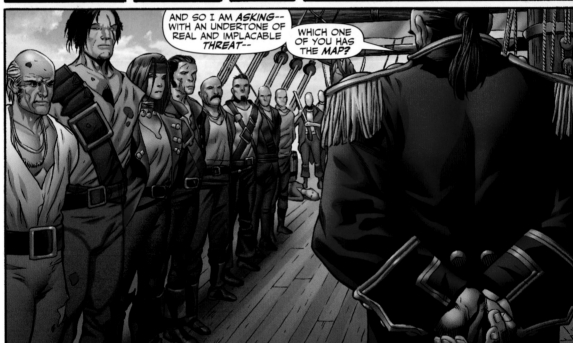

AND SO I AM *ASKING*-- WITH AN UNDERTONE OF REAL AND IMPLACABLE *THREAT*--

WHICH ONE OF YOU HAS THE *MAP*?

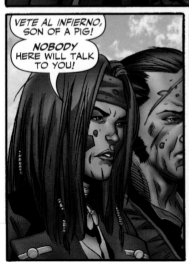

VETE AL INFIERNO, SON OF A PIG!

NOBODY HERE WILL TALK TO YOU!

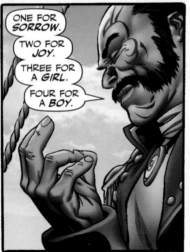

ONE FOR *SORROW*.

TWO FOR *JOY*.

THREE FOR A *GIRL*.

FOUR FOR A *BOY*.

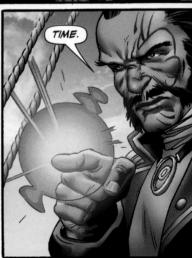

TIME.

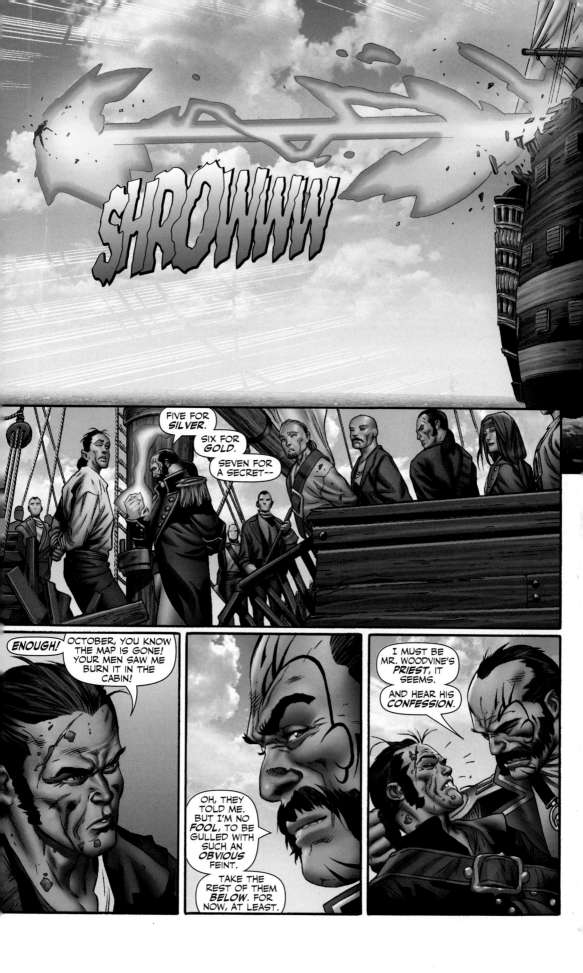

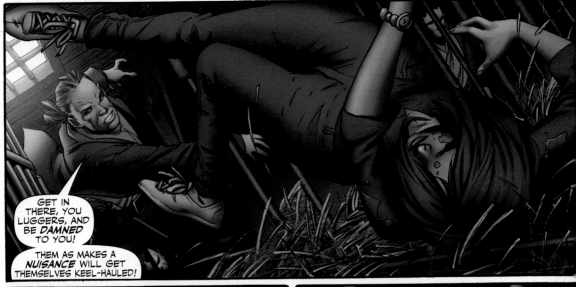

GET IN THERE, YOU LUGGERS, AND BE *DAMNED* TO YOU!

THEM AS MAKES A *NUISANCE* WILL GET THEMSELVES KEEL-HAULED!

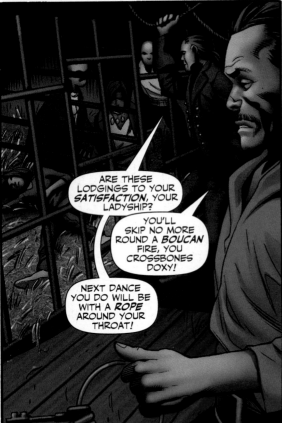

ARE THESE LODGINGS TO YOUR *SATISFACTION*, YOUR LADYSHIP?

YOU'LL SKIP NO MORE ROUND A *BOUCAN* FIRE, YOU CROSSBONES DOXY!

NEXT DANCE YOU DO WILL BE WITH A *ROPE* AROUND YOUR THROAT!

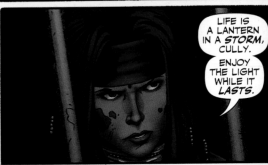

LIFE IS A LANTERN IN A *STORM*, CULLY.

ENJOY THE LIGHT WHILE IT *LASTS*.

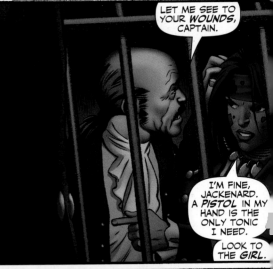

LET ME SEE TO YOUR *WOUNDS*, CAPTAIN.

I'M FINE, JACKENARD. A *PISTOL* IN MY HAND IS THE ONLY TONIC I NEED.

LOOK TO THE *GIRL*.

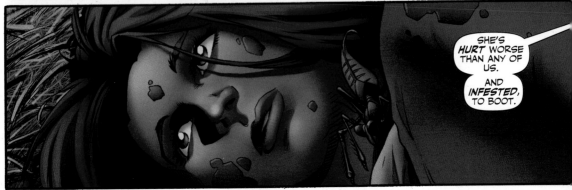

SHE'S *HURT* WORSE THAN ANY OF US.

AND *INFESTED*, TO BOOT.

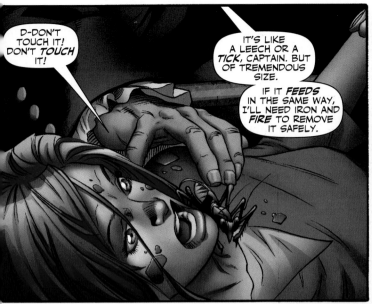

D-DON'T TOUCH IT! DON'T *TOUCH* IT!

IT'S LIKE A LEECH OR A *TICK*, CAPTAIN. BUT OF TREMENDOUS SIZE. IF IT *FEEDS* IN THE SAME WAY, I'LL NEED IRON AND *FIRE* TO REMOVE IT SAFELY.

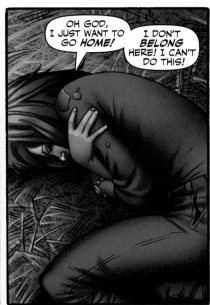

OH GOD, I JUST WANT TO GO *HOME!*

I DON'T *BELONG* HERE! I CAN'T DO THIS!

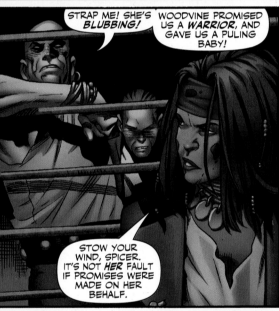

STRAP ME! SHE'S *BLUBBING!* WOODVINE PROMISED US A *WARRIOR*, AND GAVE US A PULING BABY!

STOW YOUR WIND, SPICER. IT'S NOT *HER* FAULT IF PROMISES WERE MADE ON HER BEHALF.

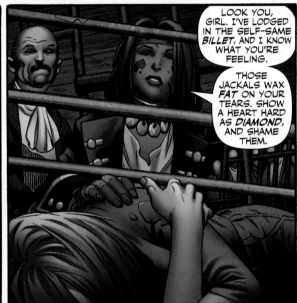

LOOK YOU, GIRL. I'VE LODGED IN THE SELF-SAME *BILLET*, AND I KNOW WHAT YOU'RE FEELING.

THOSE JACKALS WAX *FAT* ON YOUR TEARS. SHOW A HEART HARD AS *DIAMOND*, AND SHAME THEM.

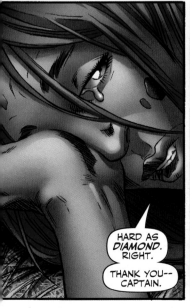

HARD AS *DIAMOND*. RIGHT.

THANK YOU-- CAPTAIN.

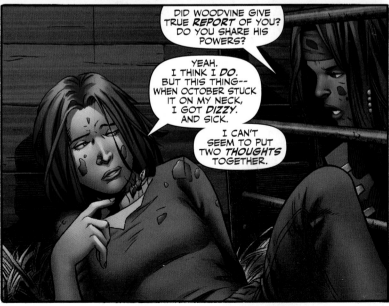

DID WOODVINE GIVE TRUE *REPORT* OF YOU? DO YOU SHARE HIS POWERS?

YEAH. I THINK I *DO*-- BUT THIS THING-- WHEN OCTOBER STUCK IT ON MY NECK, I GOT *DIZZY* AND SICK.

I CAN'T SEEM TO PUT TWO *THOUGHTS* TOGETHER.

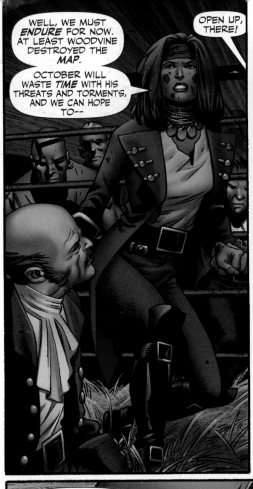

WELL, WE MUST *ENDURE* FOR NOW. AT LEAST WOODVINE DESTROYED THE *MAP*.

OCTOBER WILL WASTE *TIME* WITH HIS THREATS AND TORMENTS, AND WE CAN HOPE TO--

OPEN UP, THERE!

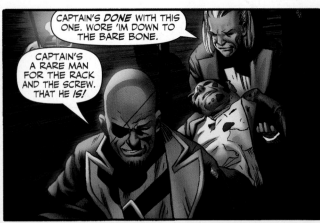

CAPTAIN'S *DONE* WITH THIS ONE. WORE 'IM DOWN TO THE BARE BONE.

CAPTAIN'S A RARE MAN FOR THE RACK AND THE SCREW. THAT HE *IS*!

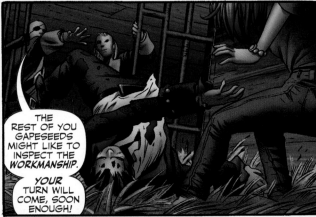

THE REST OF YOU GAPESEEDS MIGHT LIKE TO INSPECT THE *WORKMANSHIP*.

YOUR TURN WILL COME, SOON ENOUGH!

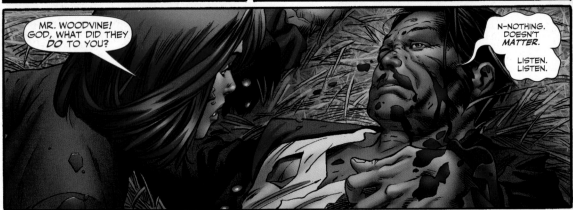

MR. WOODVINE! GOD, WHAT DID THEY *DO* TO YOU?

N-NOTHING. DOESN'T *MATTER*.

LISTEN. LISTEN.

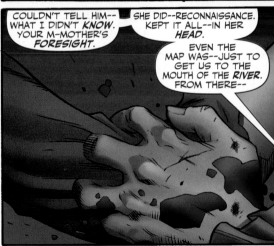

COULDN'T TELL HIM-- WHAT I DIDN'T *KNOW*. YOUR M-MOTHER'S *FORESIGHT*.

SHE DID--RECONNAISSANCE. KEPT IT ALL--IN HER *HEAD*.

EVEN THE MAP WAS--JUST TO GET US TO THE MOUTH OF THE *RIVER*. FROM THERE--

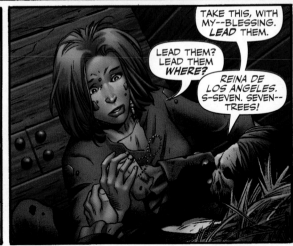

TAKE THIS, WITH MY--BLESSING. *LEAD* THEM.

LEAD THEM? LEAD THEM *WHERE*?

REINA DE LOS ANGELES. S-SEVEN. SEVEN-- TREES!

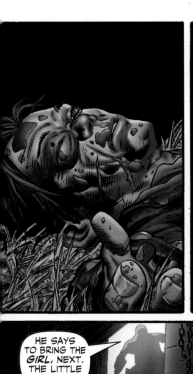
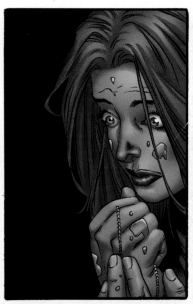
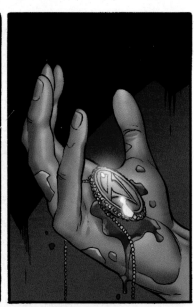

HE SAYS TO BRING THE *GIRL*, NEXT. THE LITTLE MOPPET.

AND TO TIE HER *HANDS*, AS SHE'S SUCH A *TERMAGANT*.

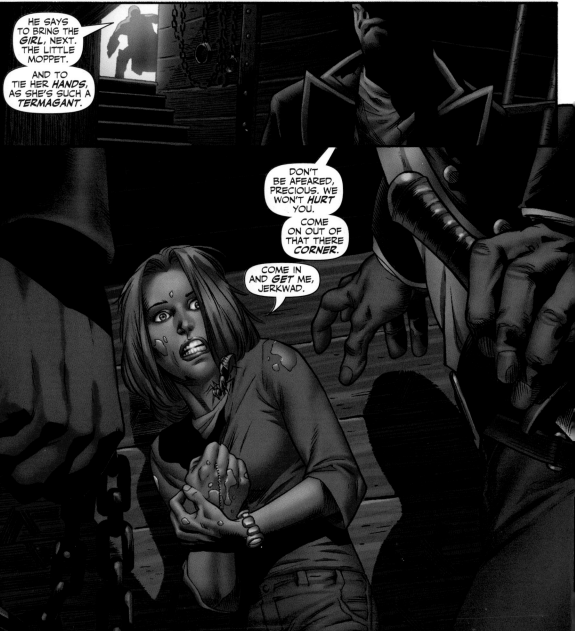

DON'T BE AFEARED, PRECIOUS. WE WON'T *HURT* YOU.

COME ON OUT OF THAT THERE *CORNER*.

COME IN AND *GET* ME, JERKWAD.

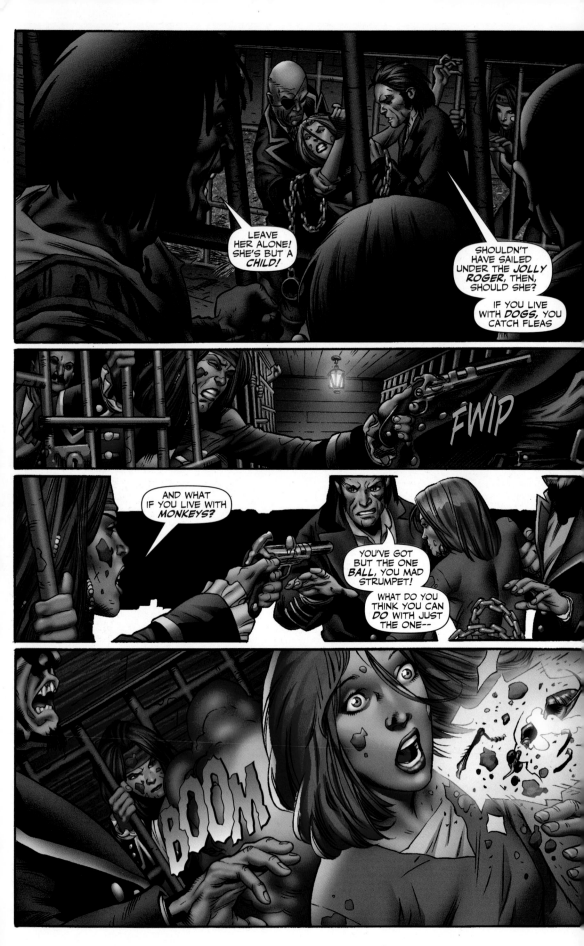

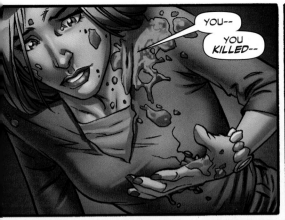

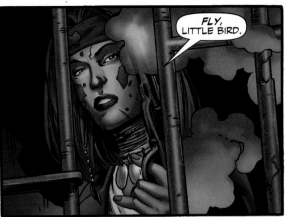

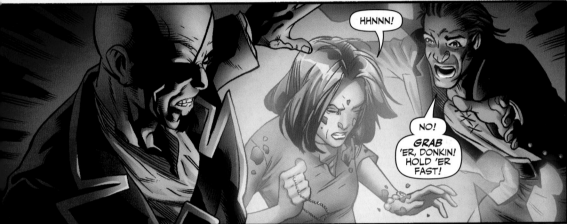

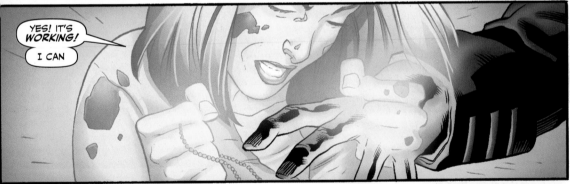

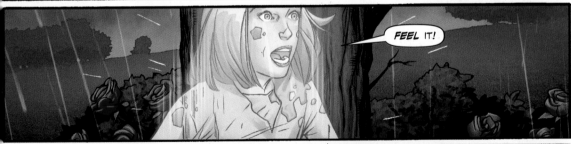

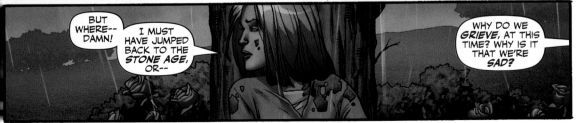

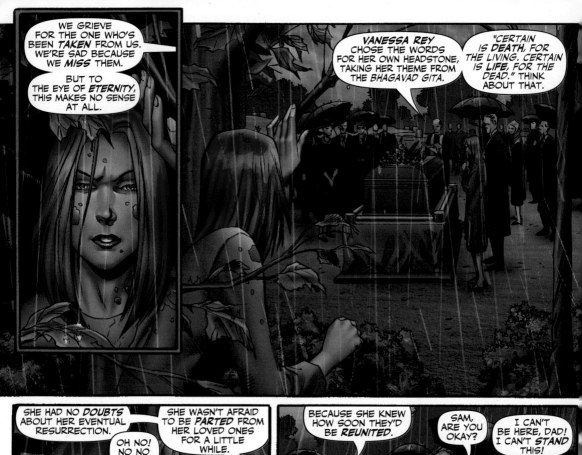

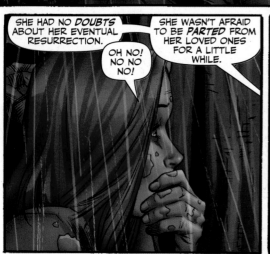

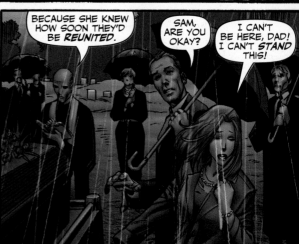

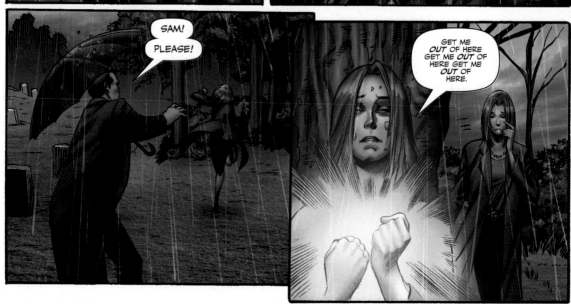

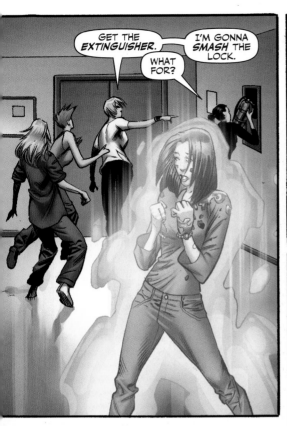
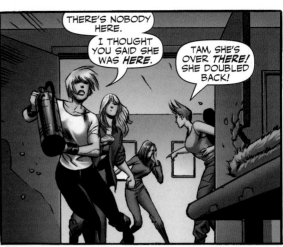
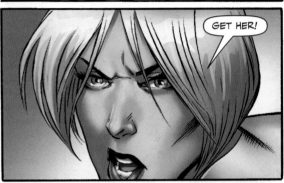
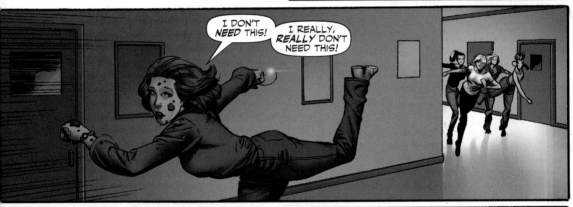
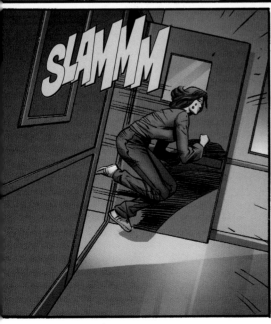
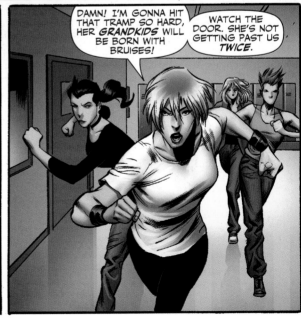

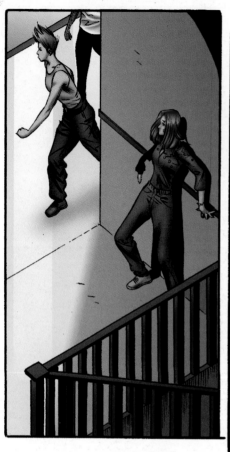
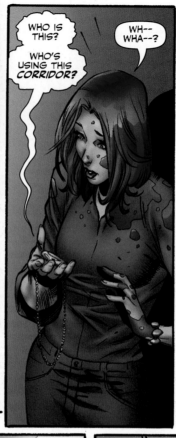
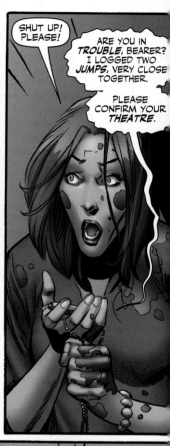
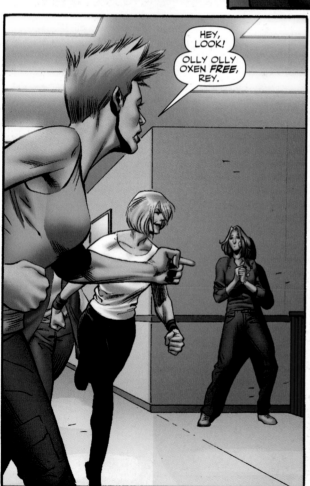
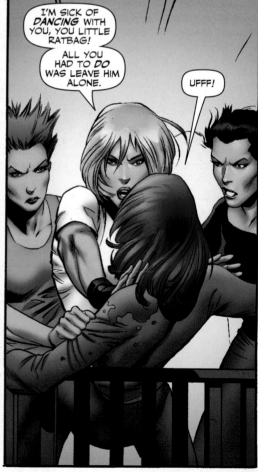

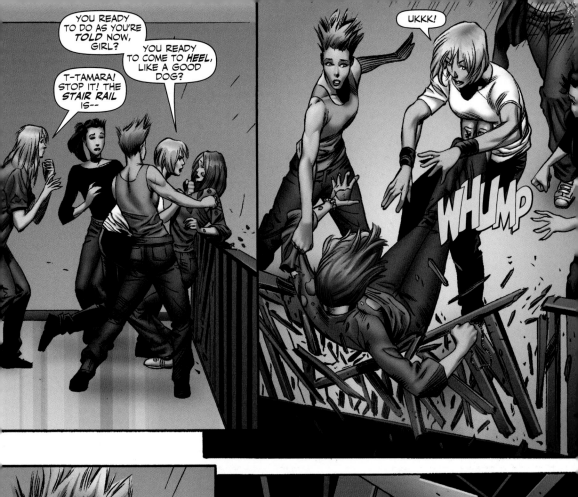
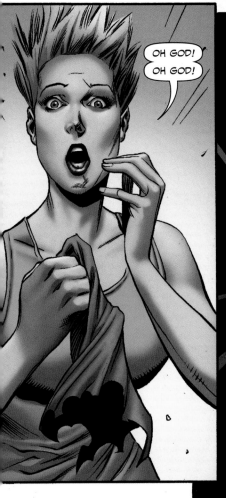
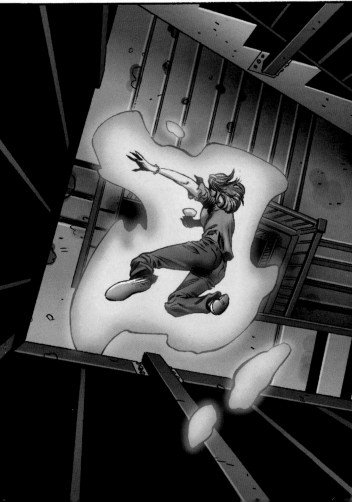

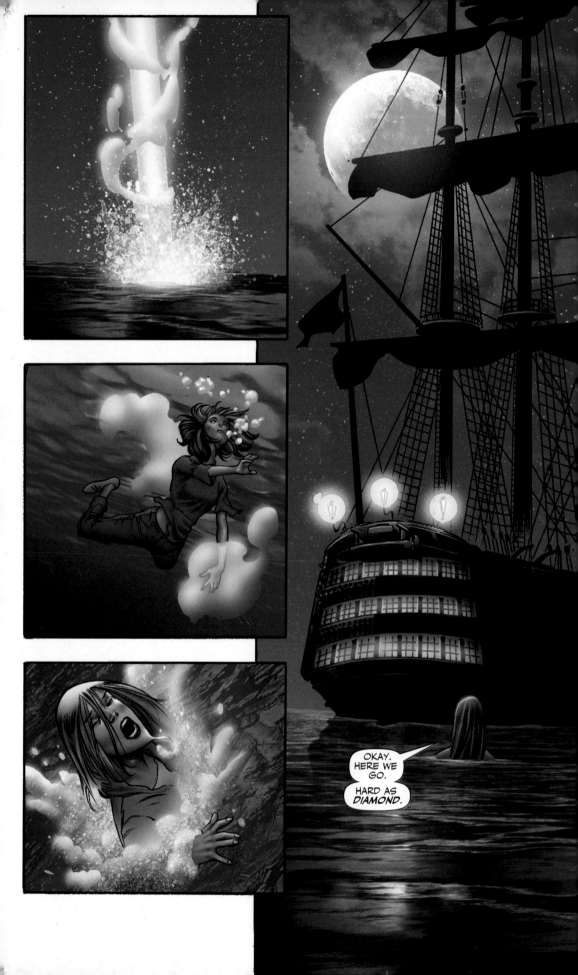

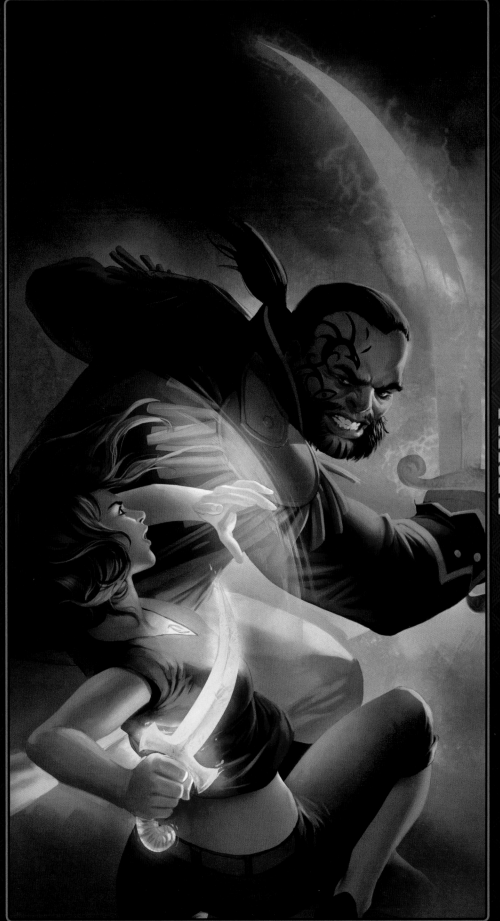

THREE

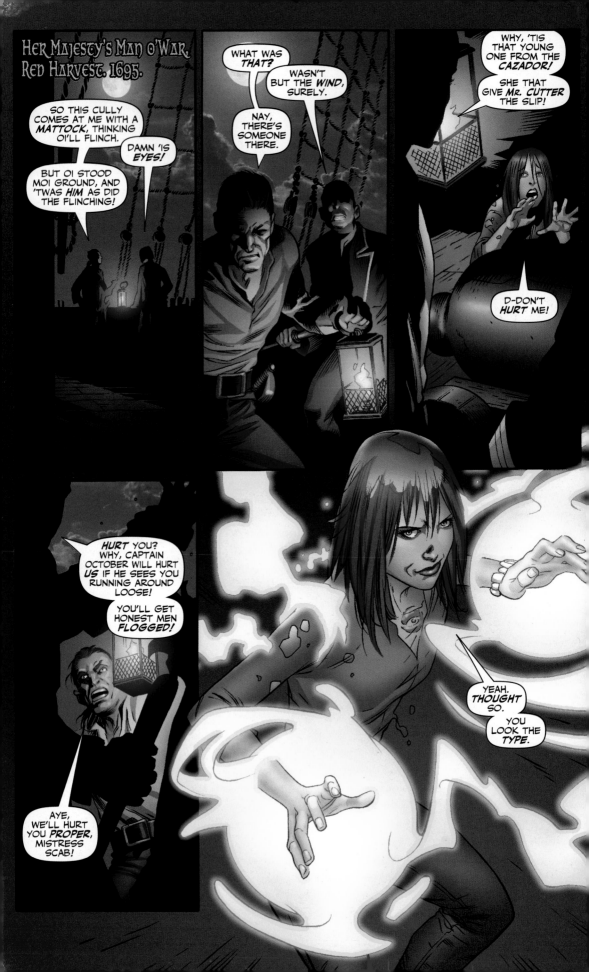

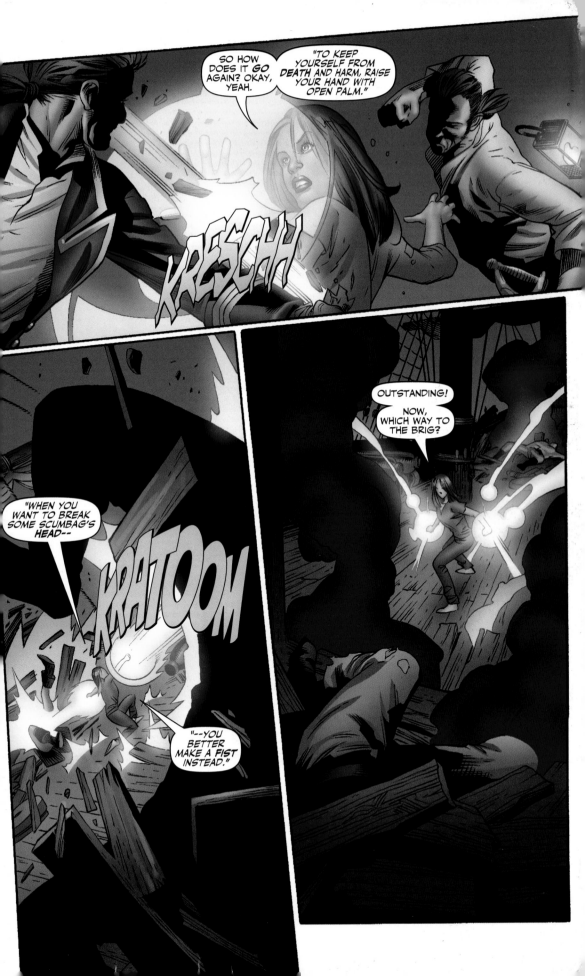

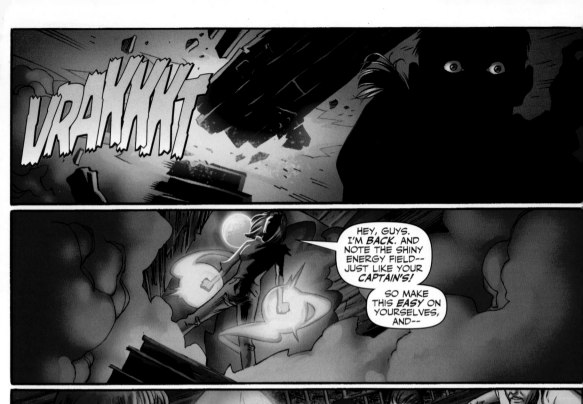

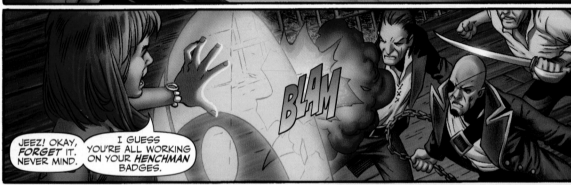

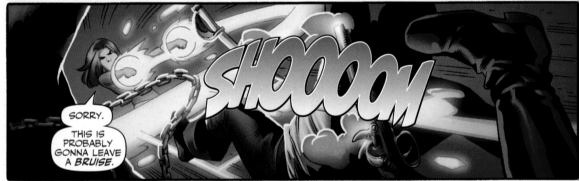

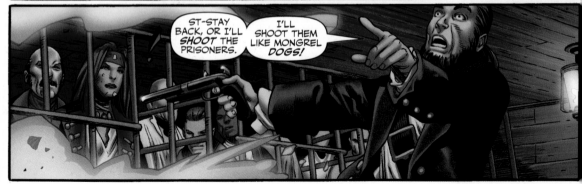

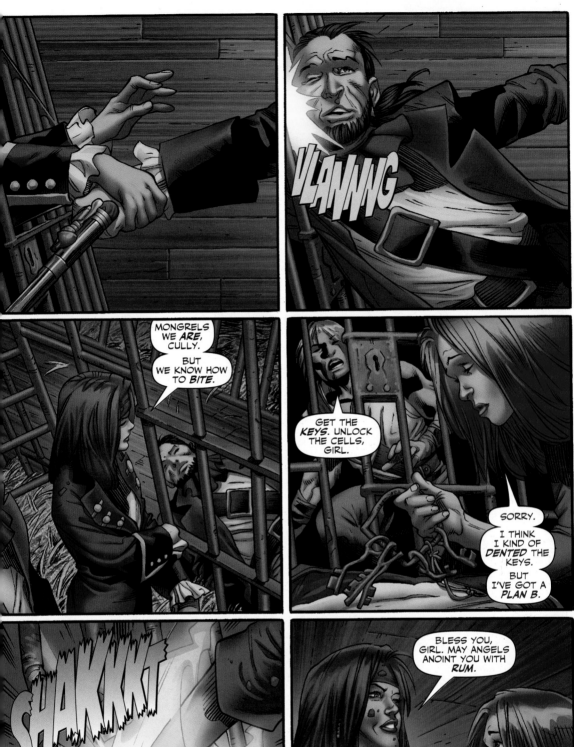

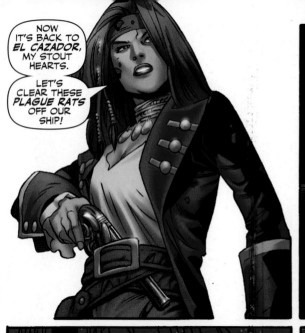

NOW IT'S BACK TO *EL CAZADOR*, MY STOUT HEARTS.

LET'S CLEAR THESE *PLAGUE RATS* OFF OUR SHIP!

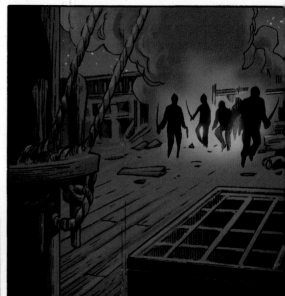

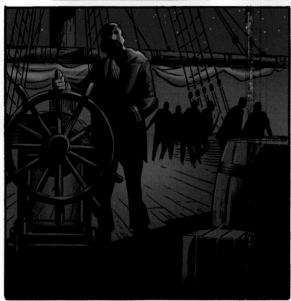

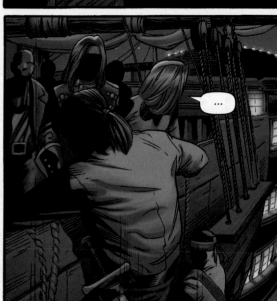

...

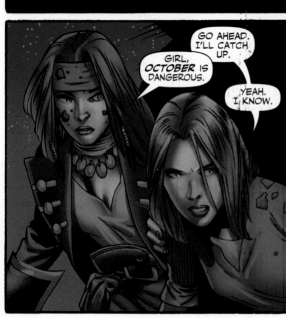

GO AHEAD. I'LL CATCH UP.

GIRL, *OCTOBER* IS DANGEROUS.

YEAH. I KNOW.

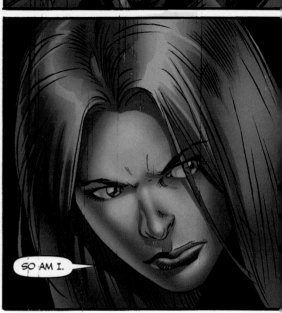

SO AM I.

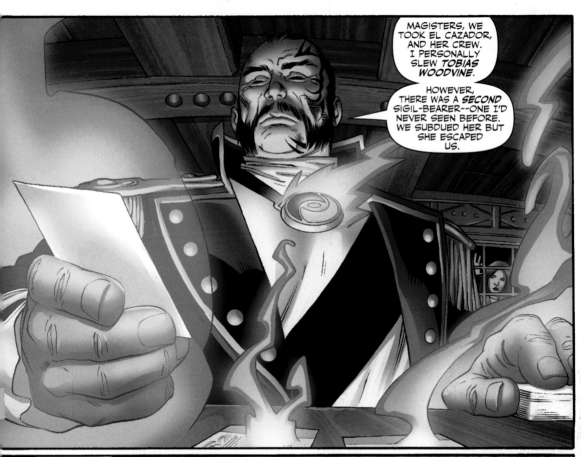

MAGISTERS, WE TOOK EL CAZADOR, AND HER CREW. I PERSONALLY SLEW *TOBIAS WOODVINE*.

HOWEVER, THERE WAS A *SECOND* SIGIL-BEARER--ONE I'D NEVER SEEN BEFORE. WE SUBDUED HER BUT SHE ESCAPED US.

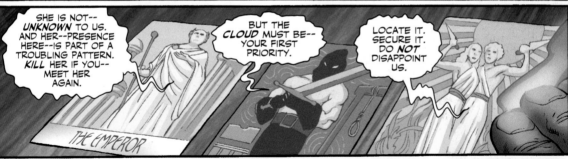

SHE IS NOT-- *UNKNOWN* TO US. AND HER--PRESENCE HERE--IS PART OF A *TROUBLING* PATTERN. *KILL* HER IF YOU-- MEET HER AGAIN.

BUT THE *CLOUD* MUST BE-- YOUR FIRST PRIORITY.

LOCATE IT. SECURE IT. DO *NOT* DISAPPOINT US.

THE EMPEROR

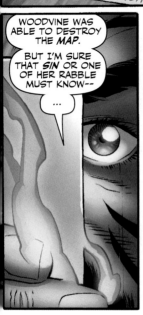

WOODVINE WAS ABLE TO DESTROY THE *MAP*.

BUT I'M SURE THAT *SIN* OR ONE OF HER RABBLE MUST KNOW--

...

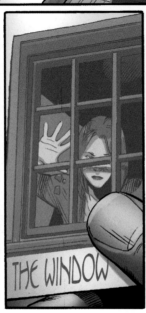

THE WINDOW

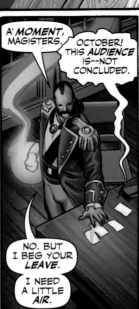

A *MOMENT*, MAGISTERS.

OCTOBER! THIS *AUDIENCE* IS--NOT CONCLUDED.

NO. BUT I BEG YOUR *LEAVE*.

I NEED A LITTLE *AIR*.

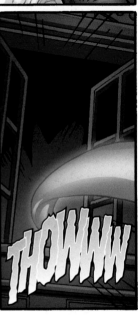

THOWWW

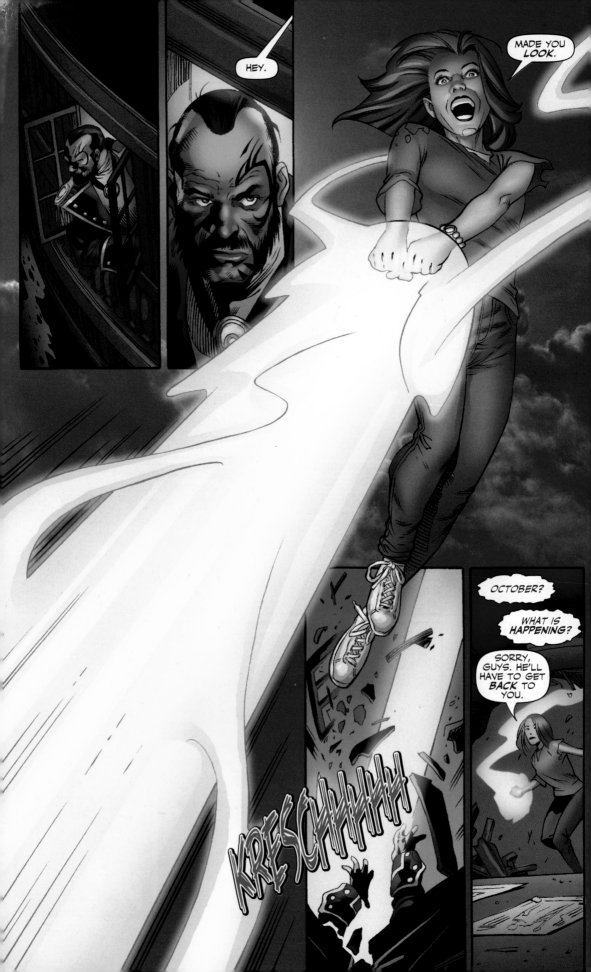

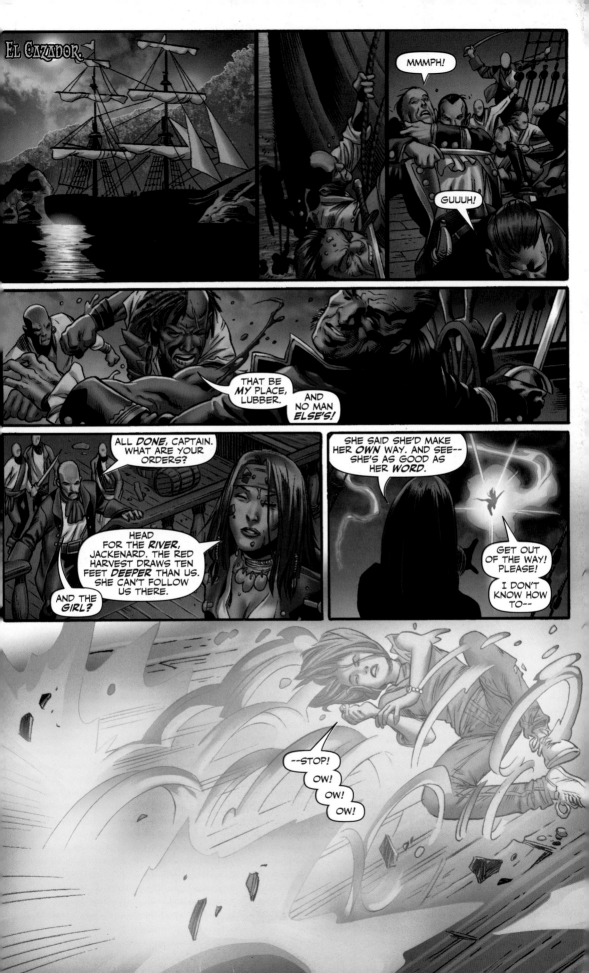

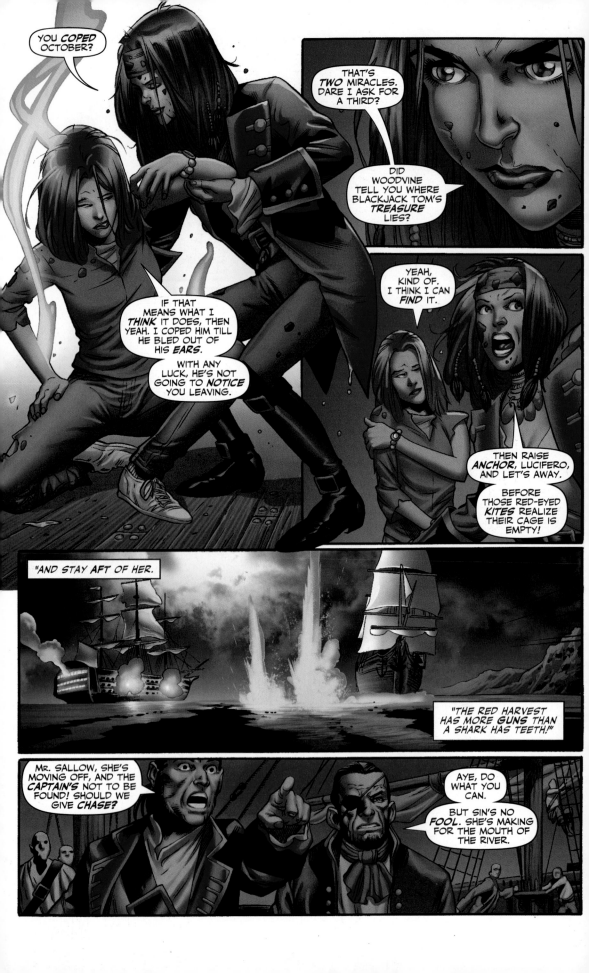

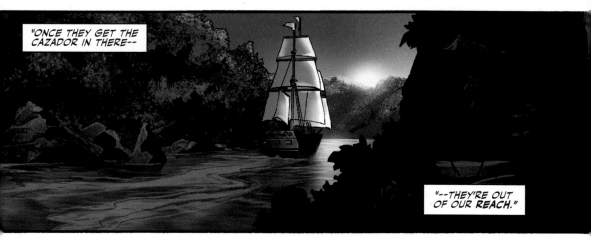

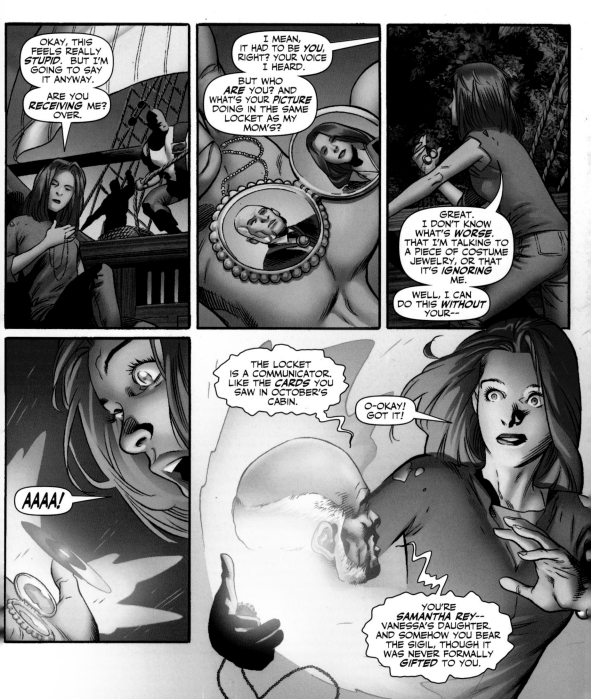

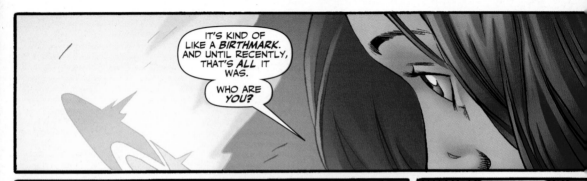

IT'S KIND OF LIKE A *BIRTHMARK.* AND UNTIL RECENTLY, THAT'S *ALL* IT WAS.

WHO ARE *YOU?*

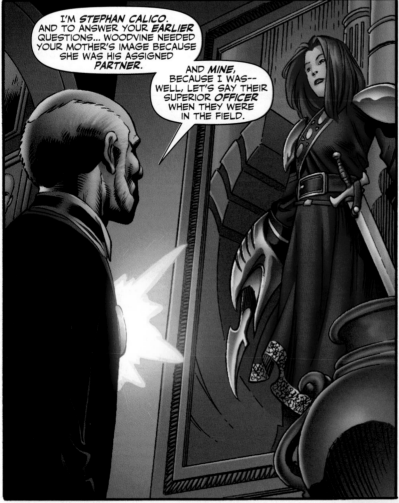

I'M *STEPHAN CALICO.* AND TO ANSWER YOUR *EARLIER* QUESTIONS... WOODVINE NEEDED YOUR MOTHER'S IMAGE BECAUSE SHE WAS HIS ASSIGNED *PARTNER.*

AND *MINE,* BECAUSE I WAS-- WELL, LET'S SAY THEIR SUPERIOR *OFFICER* WHEN THEY WERE IN THE FIELD.

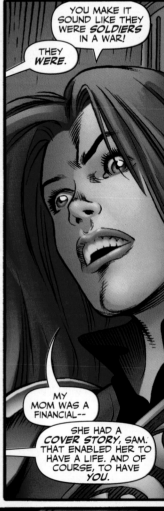

YOU MAKE IT SOUND LIKE THEY WERE *SOLDIERS* IN A WAR!

THEY *WERE.*

MY MOM WAS A FINANCIAL--

SHE HAD A *COVER STORY,* SAM. THAT ENABLED HER TO HAVE A LIFE. AND OF COURSE, TO HAVE *YOU.*

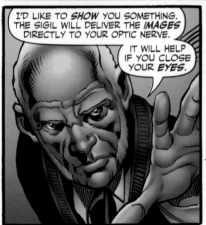

I'D LIKE TO *SHOW* YOU SOMETHING. THE SIGIL WILL DELIVER THE *IMAGES* DIRECTLY TO YOUR OPTIC NERVE.

IT WILL HELP IF YOU CLOSE YOUR *EYES.*

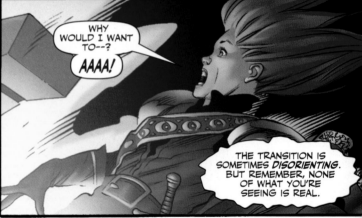

WHY WOULD I WANT TO--?

AAAA!

THE TRANSITION IS SOMETIMES *DISORIENTING.* BUT REMEMBER, NONE OF WHAT YOU'RE SEEING IS REAL.

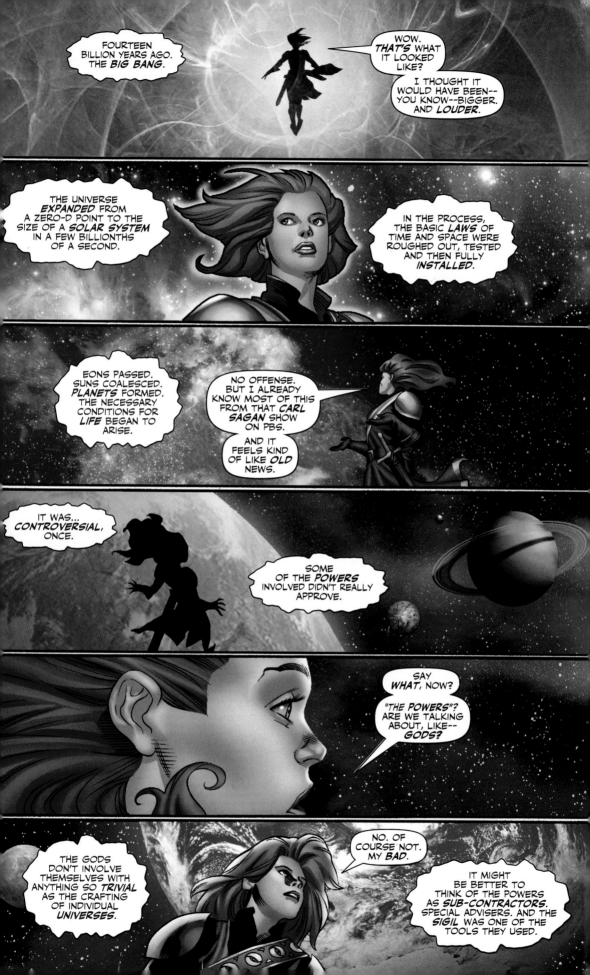

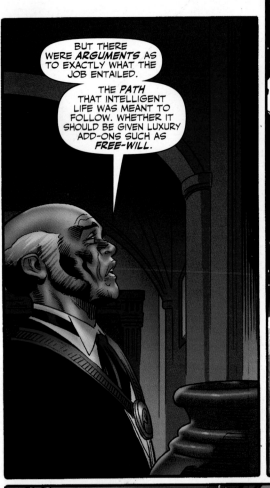

BUT THERE WERE *ARGUMENTS* AS TO EXACTLY WHAT THE JOB ENTAILED.

THE *PATH* THAT INTELLIGENT LIFE WAS MEANT TO FOLLOW. WHETHER IT SHOULD BE GIVEN LUXURY ADD-ONS SUCH AS *FREE-WILL*.

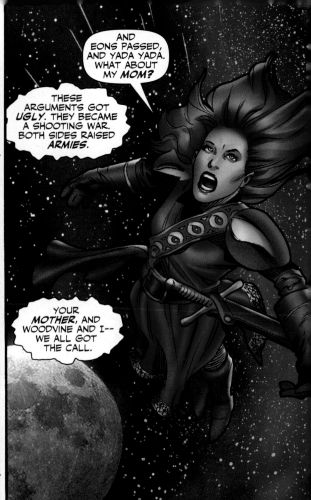

AND EONS PASSED, AND YADA YADA. WHAT ABOUT MY *MOM?*

THESE ARGUMENTS GOT *UGLY*. THEY BECAME A SHOOTING WAR. BOTH SIDES RAISED *ARMIES*.

YOUR *MOTHER*, AND WOODVINE AND I-- WE ALL GOT THE CALL.

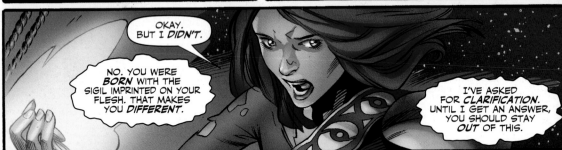

OKAY. BUT I *DIDN'T.*

NO. YOU WERE *BORN* WITH THE SIGIL IMPRINTED ON YOUR FLESH. THAT MAKES YOU *DIFFERENT.*

I'VE ASKED FOR *CLARIFICATION.* UNTIL I GET AN ANSWER, YOU SHOULD STAY *OUT* OF THIS.

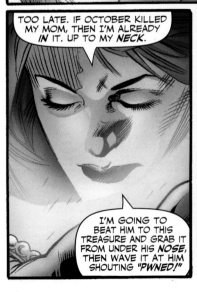

TOO LATE. IF OCTOBER KILLED MY MOM, THEN I'M ALREADY *IN* IT. UP TO MY *NECK.*

I'M GOING TO BEAT HIM TO THIS TREASURE AND GRAB IT FROM UNDER HIS *NOSE*, THEN WAVE IT AT HIM SHOUTING *"PWNED!"*

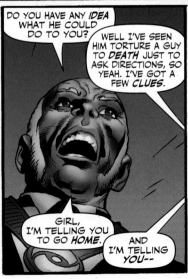

DO YOU HAVE ANY *IDEA* WHAT HE COULD DO TO YOU?

WELL I'VE SEEN HIM TORTURE A GUY TO *DEATH* JUST TO ASK DIRECTIONS, SO YEAH. I'VE GOT A FEW *CLUES.*

GIRL, I'M TELLING YOU TO GO *HOME.*

AND I'M TELLING *YOU*--

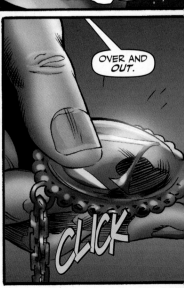

OVER AND *OUT.*

CLICK

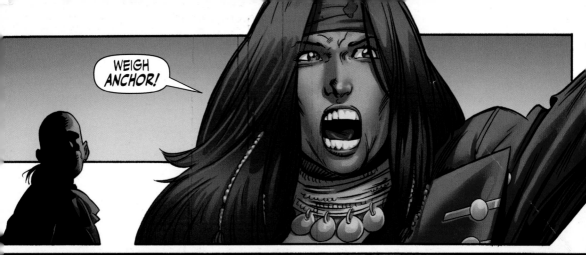

WEIGH *ANCHOR!*

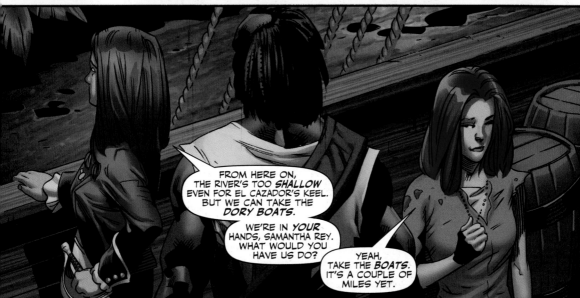

FROM HERE ON, THE RIVER'S TOO *SHALLOW* EVEN FOR EL CAZADOR'S KEEL. BUT WE CAN TAKE THE *DORY BOATS.*

WE'RE IN *YOUR* HANDS, SAMANTHA REY. WHAT WOULD YOU HAVE US DO?

YEAH, TAKE THE *BOATS.* IT'S A COUPLE OF MILES YET.

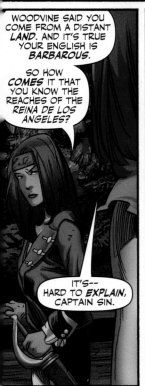

WOODVINE SAID YOU COME FROM A DISTANT *LAND.* AND IT'S TRUE YOUR ENGLISH IS *BARBAROUS.*

SO HOW *COMES* IT THAT YOU KNOW THE REACHES OF THE *REINA DE LOS ANGELES?*

IT'S-- HARD TO *EXPLAIN,* CAPTAIN SIN.

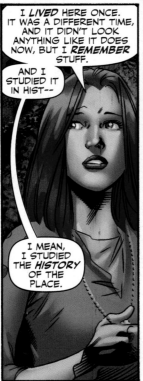

I *LIVED* HERE ONCE. IT WAS A DIFFERENT TIME, AND IT DIDN'T LOOK ANYTHING LIKE IT DOES NOW, BUT I *REMEMBER* STUFF.

AND I STUDIED IT IN HIST--

I MEAN, I STUDIED THE *HISTORY* OF THE PLACE.

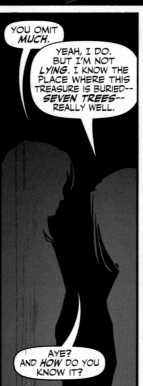

YOU OMIT *MUCH.*

YEAH, I DO. BUT I'M NOT *LYING.* I KNOW THE PLACE WHERE THIS TREASURE IS BURIED-- *SEVEN TREES--* REALLY WELL.

AYE? AND *HOW* DO YOU KNOW IT?

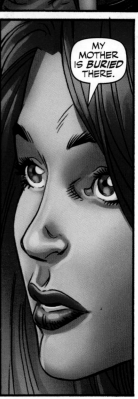

MY MOTHER IS *BURIED* THERE.

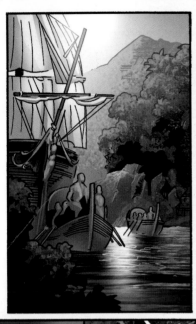

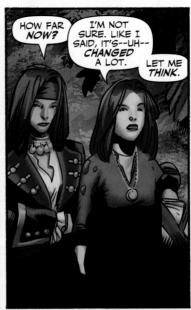

HOW FAR *NOW?*

I'M NOT SURE. LIKE I SAID, IT'S--UH-- *CHANGED* A LOT.

LET ME *THINK.*

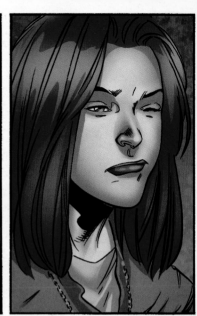

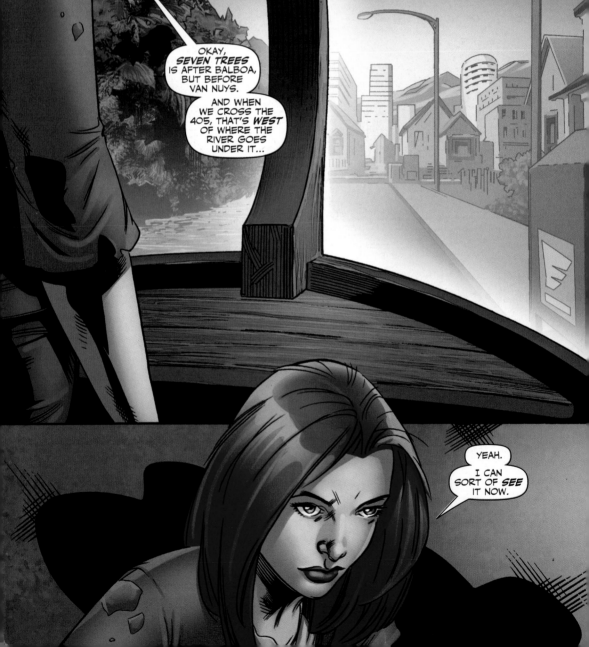

OKAY, *SEVEN TREES* IS AFTER BALBOA, BUT BEFORE VAN NUYS.

AND WHEN WE CROSS THE 405, THAT'S *WEST* OF WHERE THE RIVER GOES UNDER IT...

YEAH. I CAN SORT OF *SEE* IT NOW.

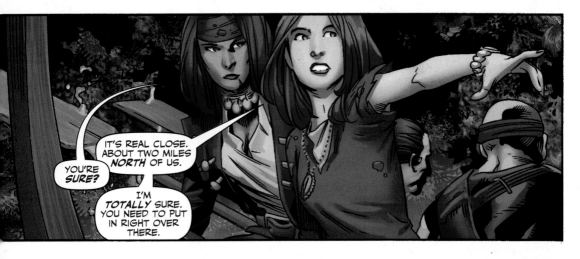

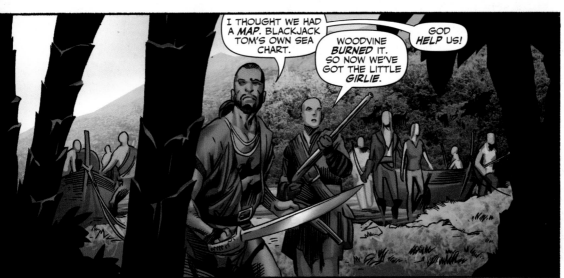

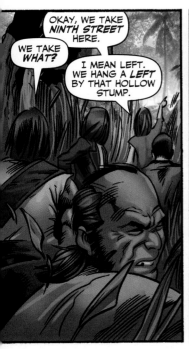

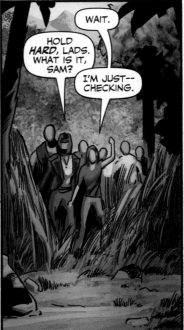

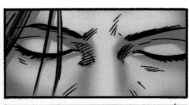

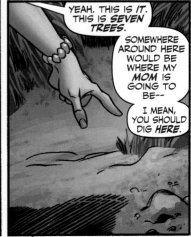

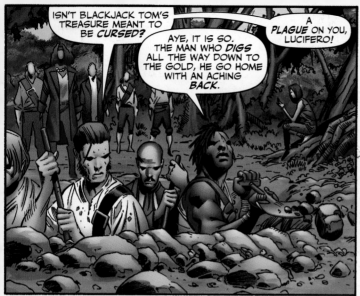

ISN'T BLACKJACK TOM'S TREASURE MEANT TO BE *CURSED?*

AYE, IT IS SO. THE MAN WHO *DIGS* ALL THE WAY DOWN TO THE GOLD, HE GO HOME WITH AN ACHING *BACK.*

A *PLAGUE* ON YOU, LUCIFERO!

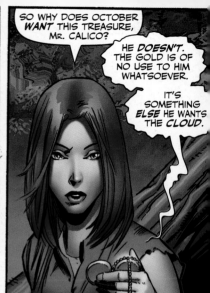

SO WHY DOES OCTOBER *WANT* THIS TREASURE, MR. CALICO?

HE *DOESN'T.* THE GOLD IS OF NO USE TO HIM WHATSOEVER.

IT'S SOMETHING *ELSE* HE WANTS THE *CLOUD.*

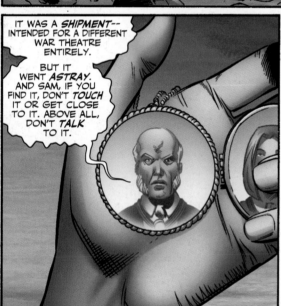

IT WAS A *SHIPMENT--* INTENDED FOR A DIFFERENT WAR THEATRE ENTIRELY.

BUT IT WENT *ASTRAY.* AND SAM, IF YOU FIND IT, DON'T *TOUCH* IT OR GET CLOSE TO IT. ABOVE ALL, DON'T *TALK* TO IT.

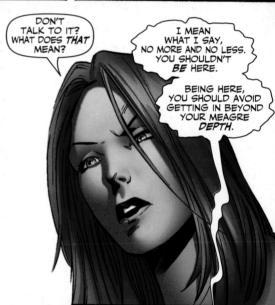

DON'T TALK TO IT? WHAT DOES *THAT* MEAN?

I MEAN WHAT I SAY, NO MORE AND NO LESS. YOU SHOULDN'T *BE* HERE.

BEING HERE, YOU SHOULD AVOID GETTING IN BEYOND YOUR MEAGRE *DEPTH.*

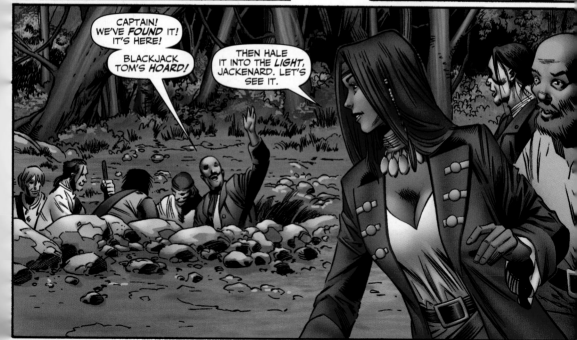

CAPTAIN! WE'VE *FOUND* IT! IT'S HERE!

BLACKJACK TOM'S *HOARD!*

THEN HALE IT INTO THE *LIGHT,* JACKENARD. LET'S SEE IT.

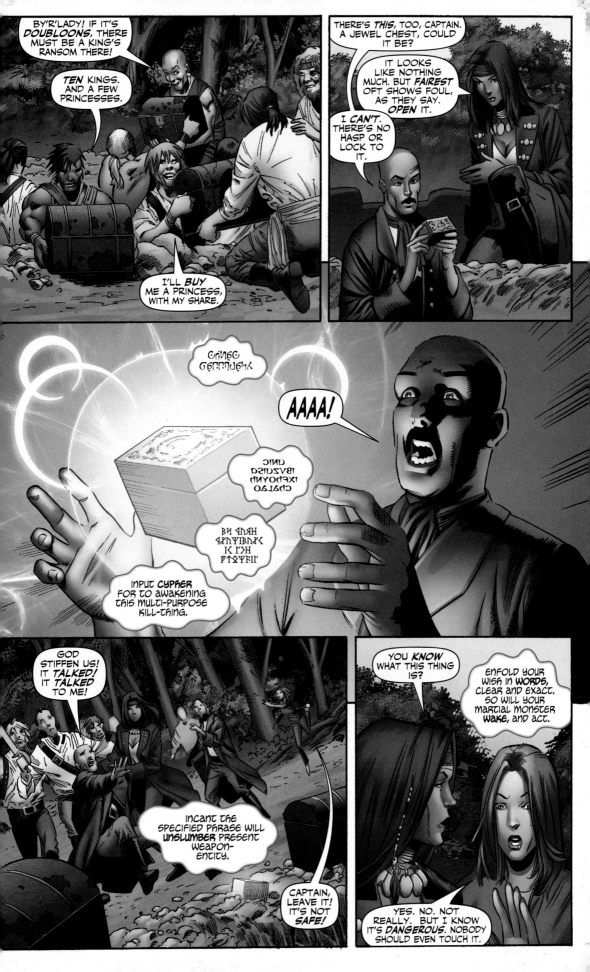

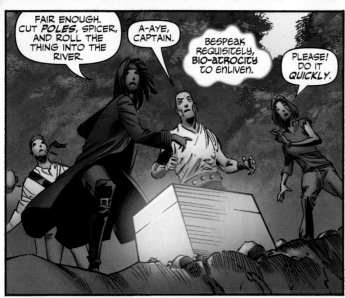

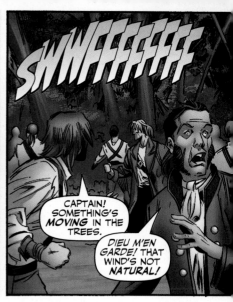

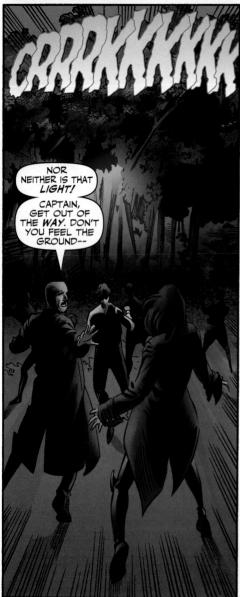

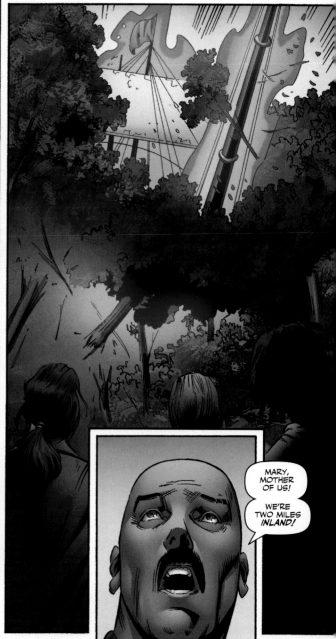

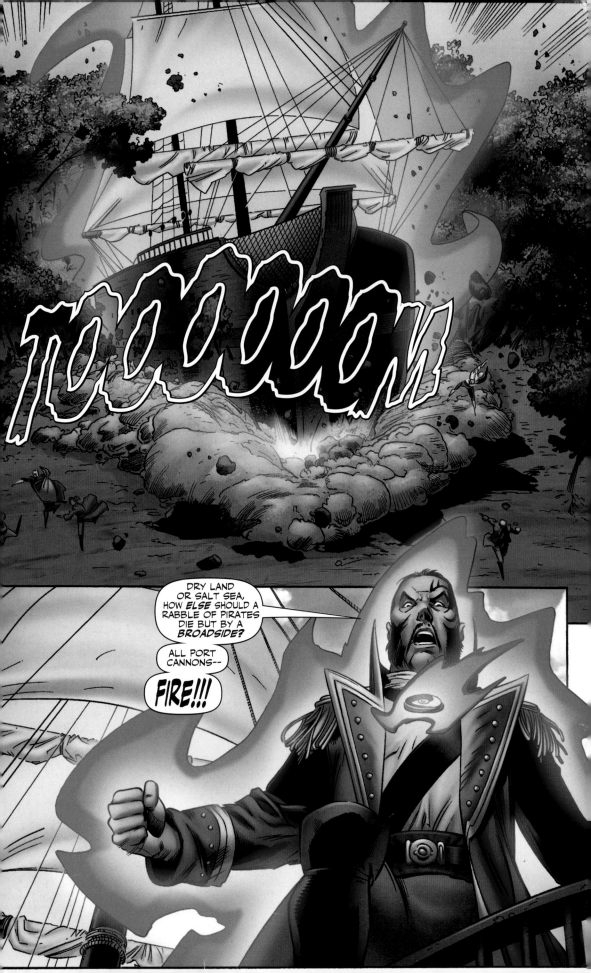

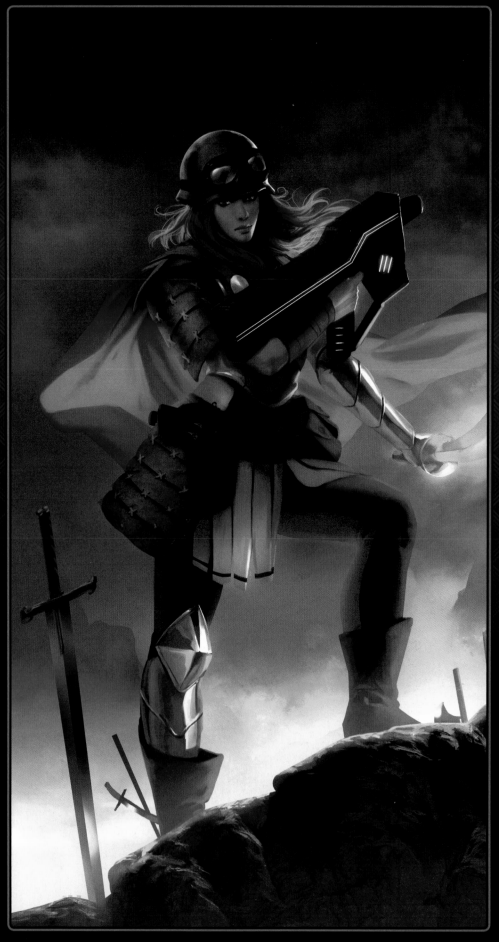

FOUR

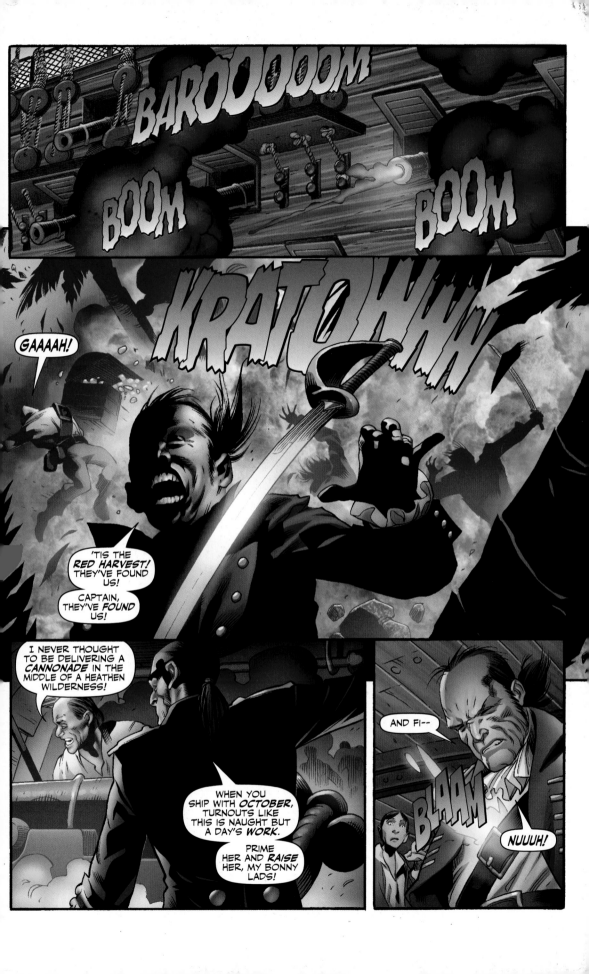

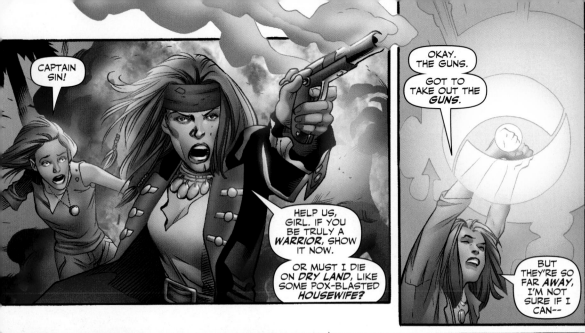

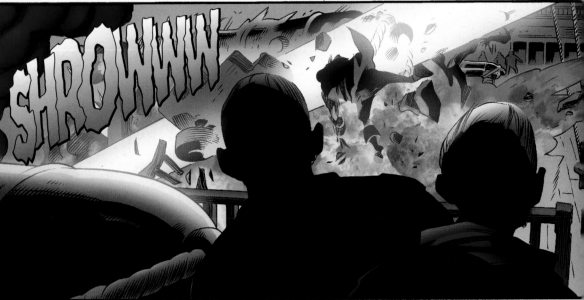

SHROWNN

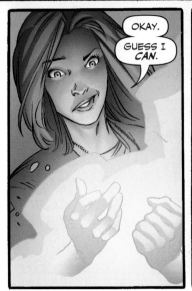

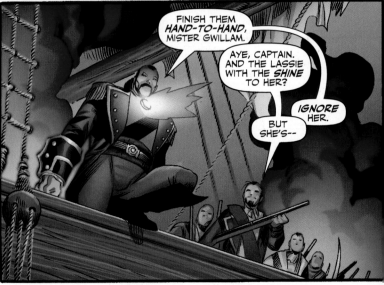

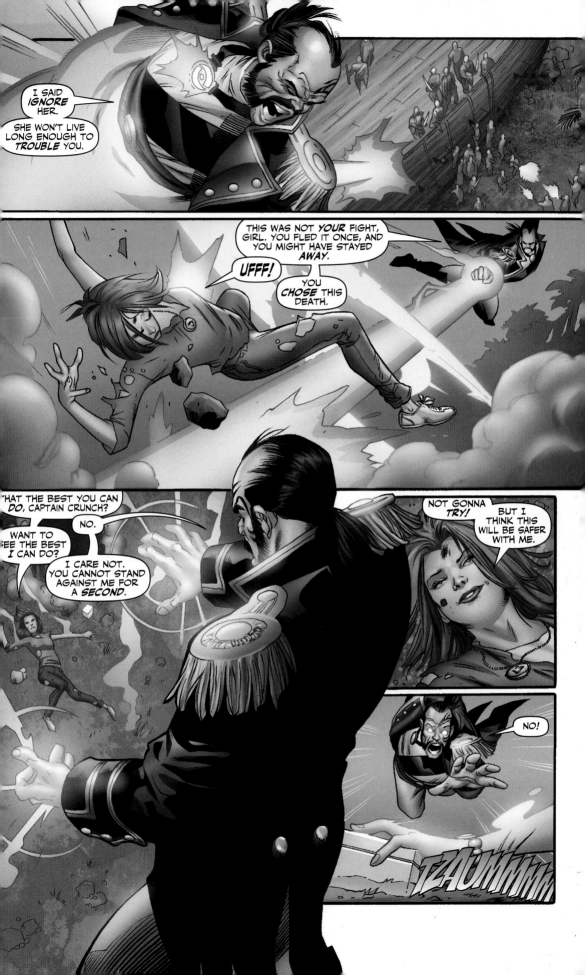

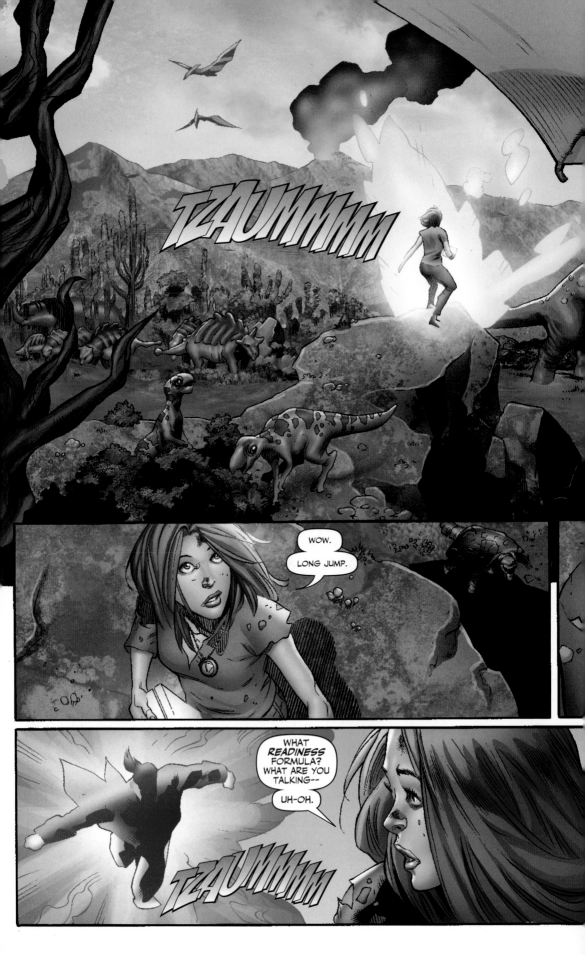

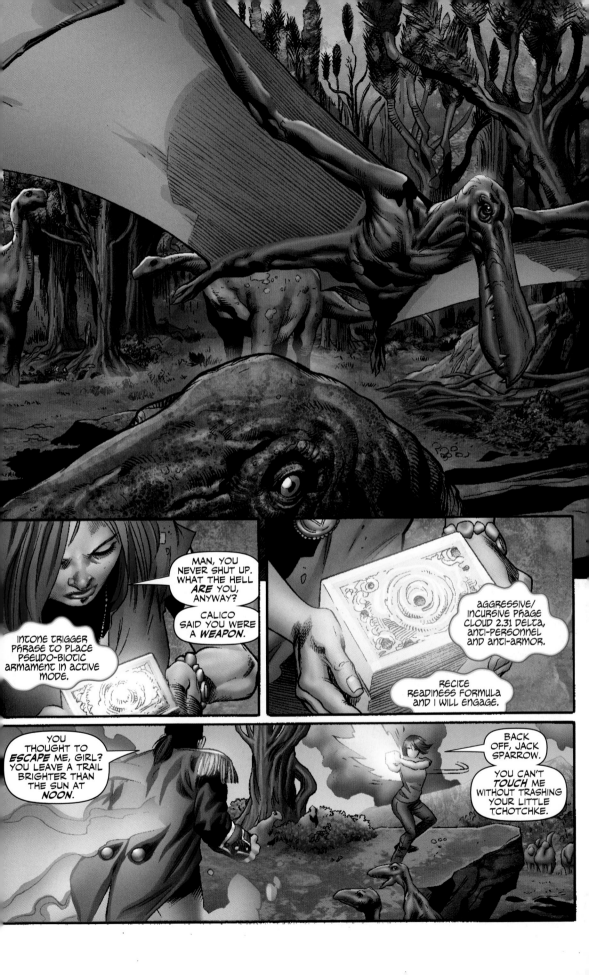

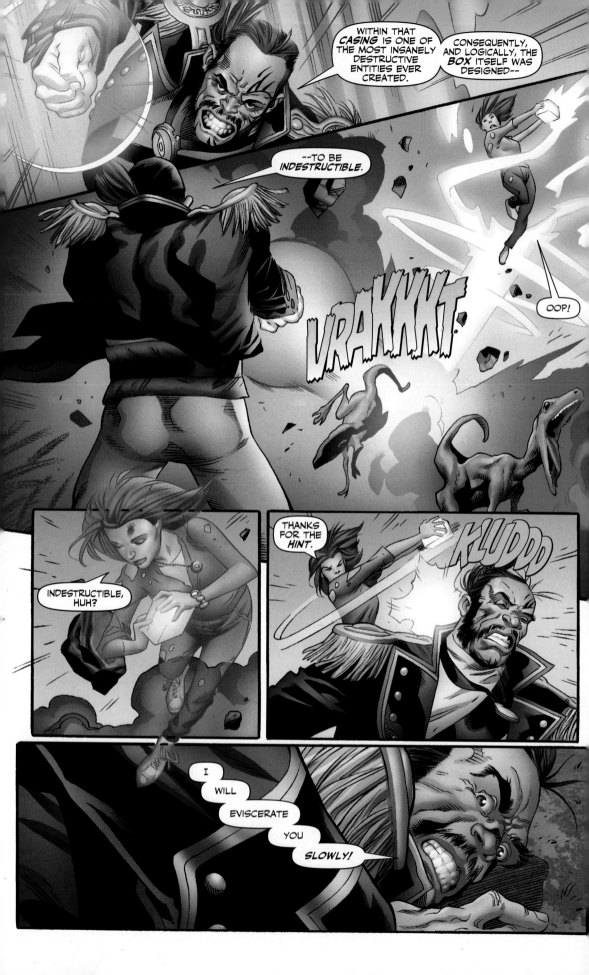

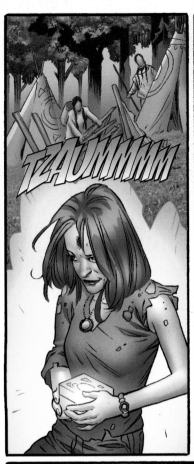

TZAUMMMM

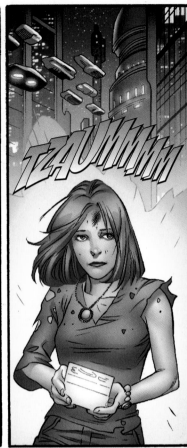

TZAUMMMM

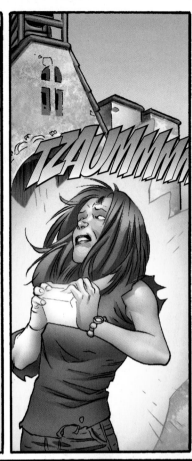

TZAUMMMM

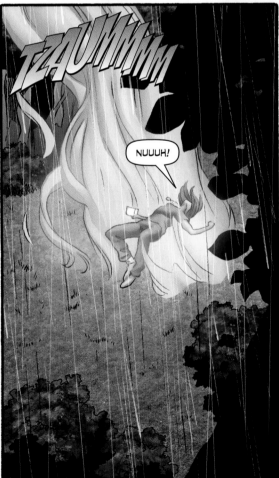

TZAUMMMM

NUUUH!

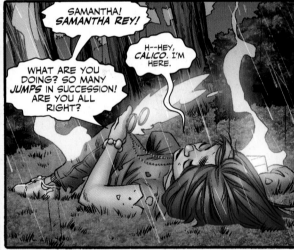

SAMANTHA! *SAMANTHA REY!*

WHAT ARE YOU DOING? SO MANY *JUMPS* IN SUCCESSION! ARE YOU ALL RIGHT?

H--HEY, *CALICO.* I'M HERE.

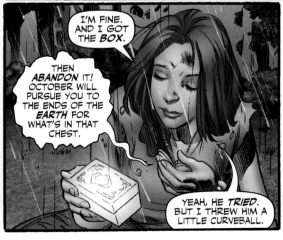

I'M FINE. AND I GOT THE *BOX.*

THEN *ABANDON* IT! OCTOBER WILL PURSUE YOU TO THE ENDS OF THE *EARTH* FOR WHAT'S IN THAT CHEST.

YEAH, HE *TRIED.* BUT I THREW HIM A LITTLE CURVEBALL.

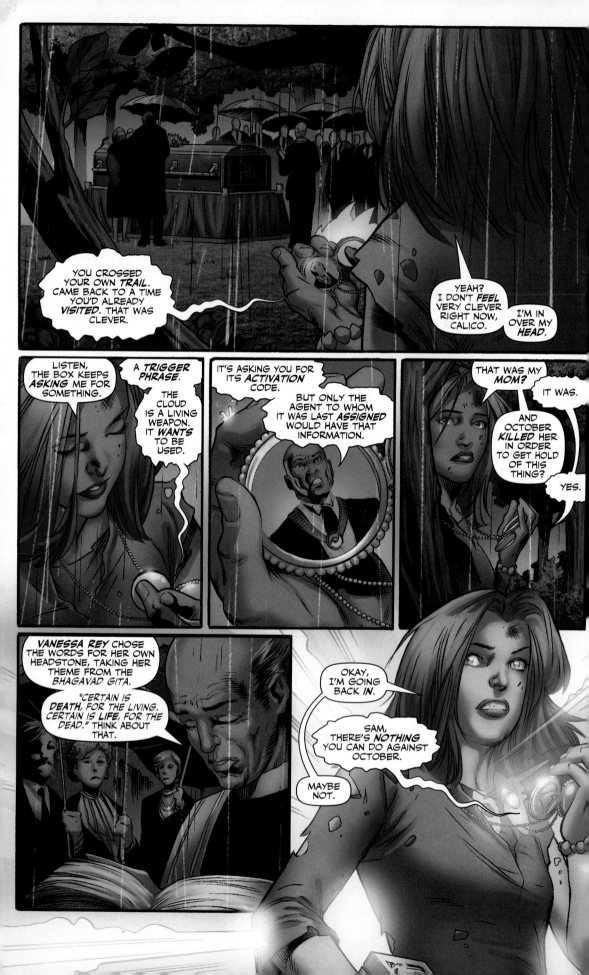

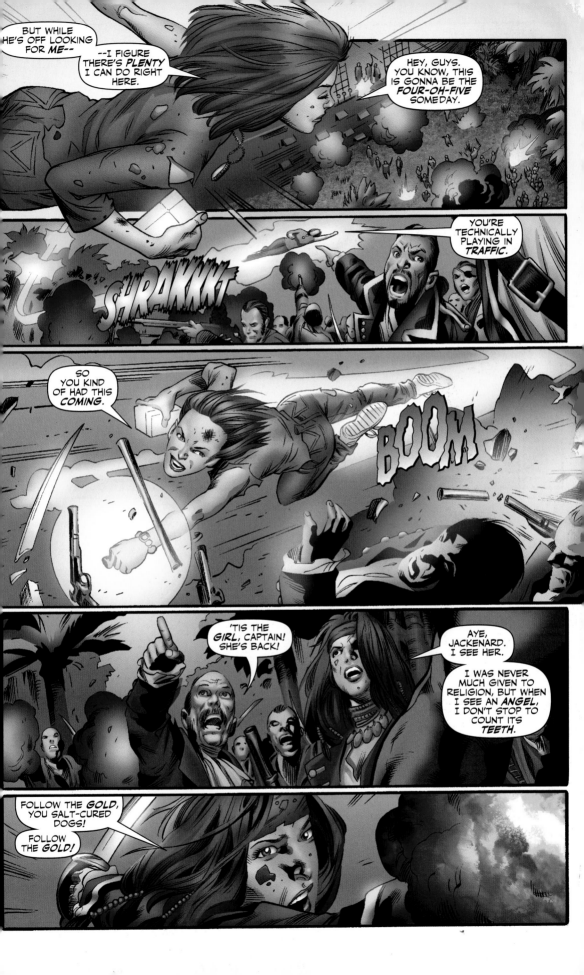

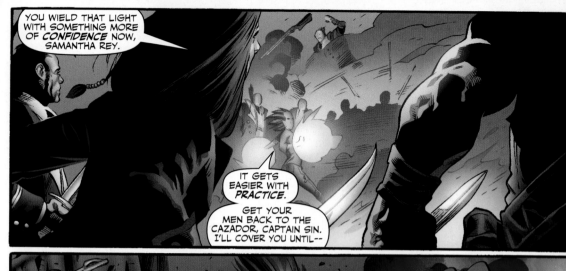

YOU WIELD THAT LIGHT WITH SOMETHING MORE OF *CONFIDENCE* NOW, SAMANTHA REY.

IT GETS EASIER WITH *PRACTICE.*

GET YOUR MEN BACK TO THE CAZADOR, CAPTAIN SIN. I'LL COVER YOU UNTIL--

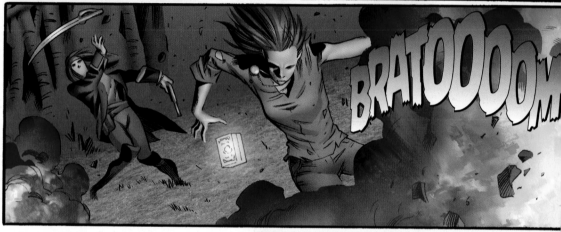

BRATOOOOM

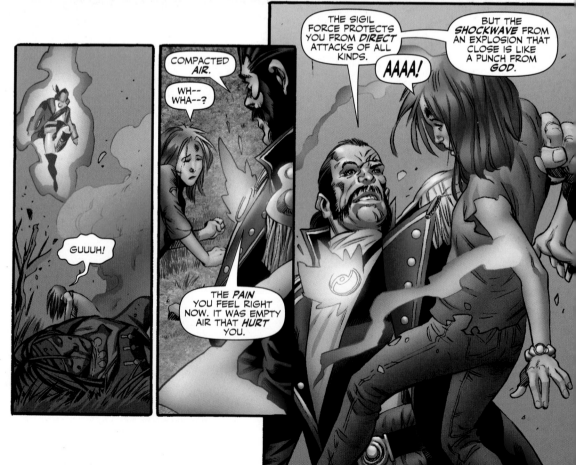

THE SIGIL FORCE PROTECTS YOU FROM *DIRECT* ATTACKS OF ALL KINDS.

BUT THE *SHOCKWAVE* FROM AN EXPLOSION THAT CLOSE IS LIKE A PUNCH FROM *GOD.*

AAAA!

COMPACTED *AIR.*

WH-- WHA--?

GUUUH!

THE *PAIN* YOU FEEL RIGHT NOW. IT WAS EMPTY AIR THAT *HURT* YOU.

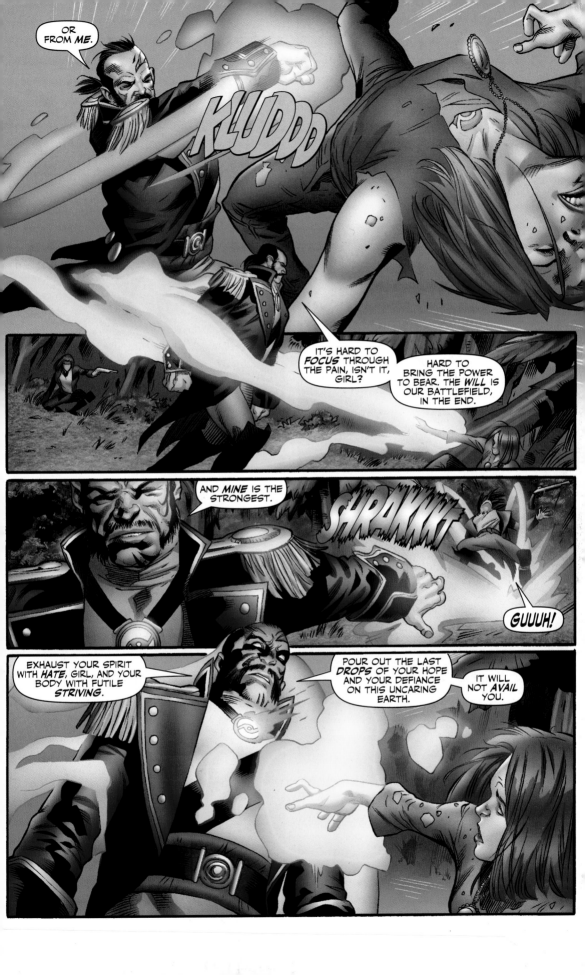

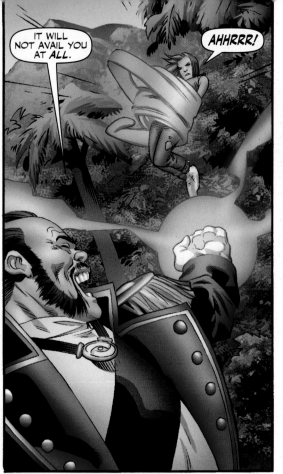

IT WILL NOT AVAIL YOU AT *ALL.*

AHHRRR!

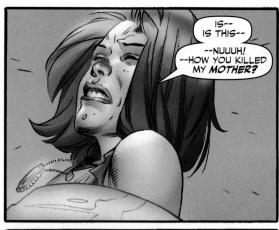

IS-- IS THIS-- --NUUUH! --HOW YOU KILLED MY *MOTHER?*

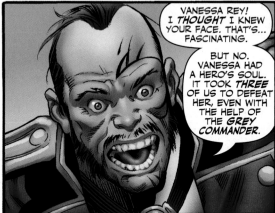

VANESSA REY! I *THOUGHT* I KNEW YOUR FACE. THAT'S... FASCINATING.

BUT NO. VANESSA HAD A HERO'S SOUL. IT TOOK *THREE* OF US TO DEFEAT HER, EVEN WITH THE HELP OF THE *GREY COMMANDER.*

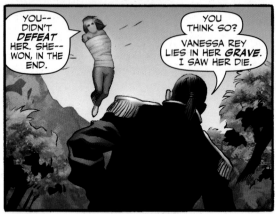

YOU-- DIDN'T *DEFEAT* HER. SHE-- WON, IN THE END.

YOU THINK SO? VANESSA REY LIES IN HER *GRAVE.* I SAW HER DIE.

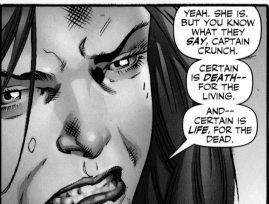

YEAH. SHE IS. BUT YOU KNOW WHAT THEY *SAY,* CAPTAIN CRUNCH.

CERTAIN IS *DEATH*-- FOR THE LIVING.

AND-- CERTAIN IS *LIFE,* FOR THE DEAD.

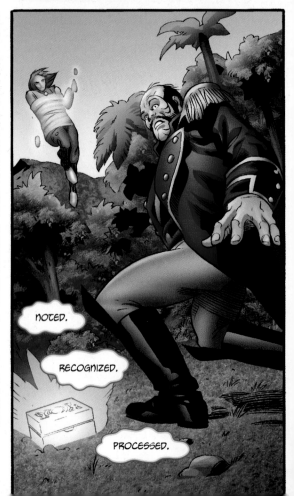

NOTED.

RECOGNIZED.

PROCESSED.

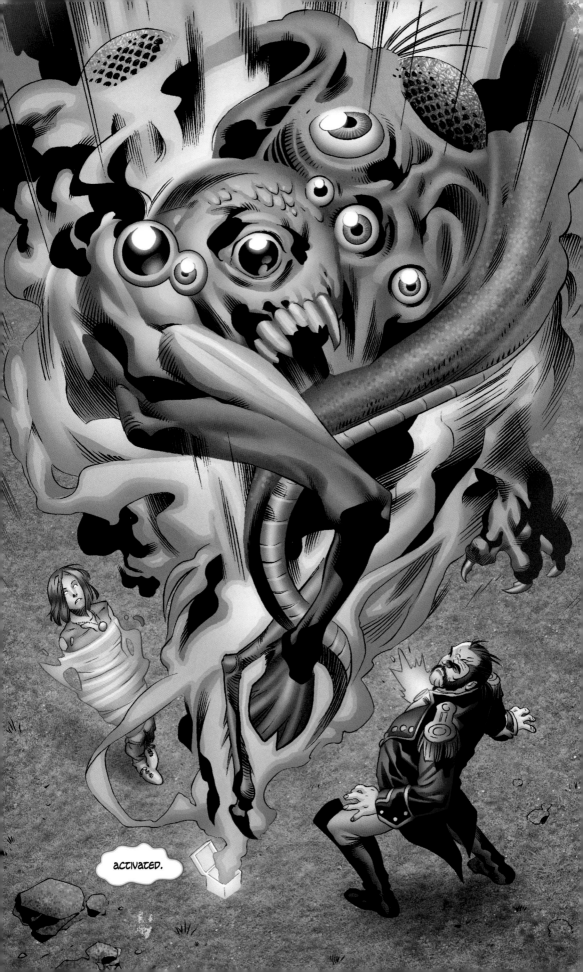

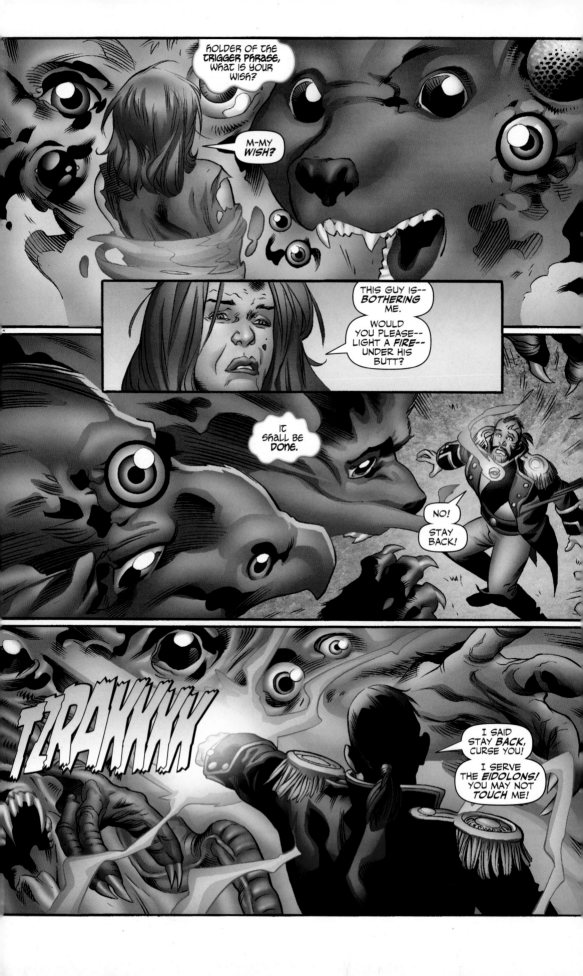

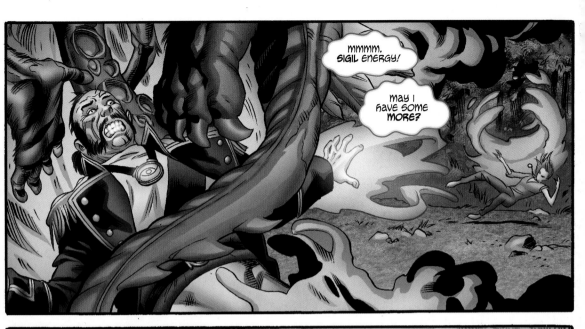
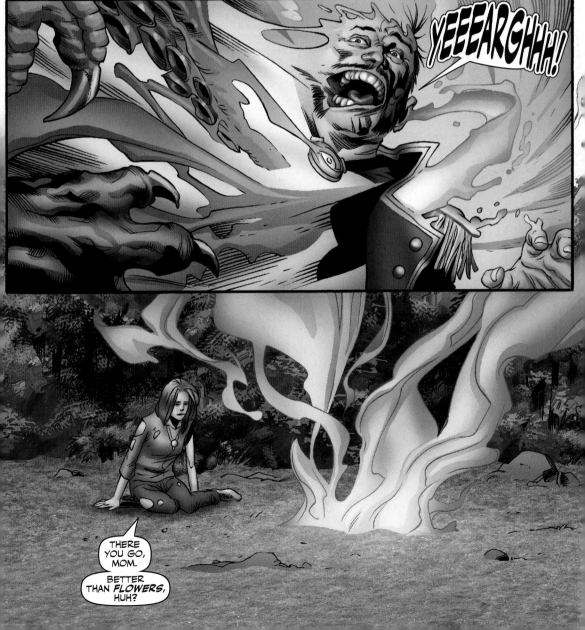

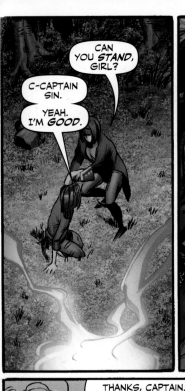

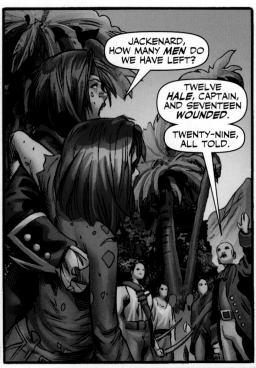

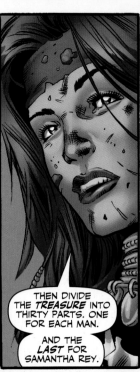

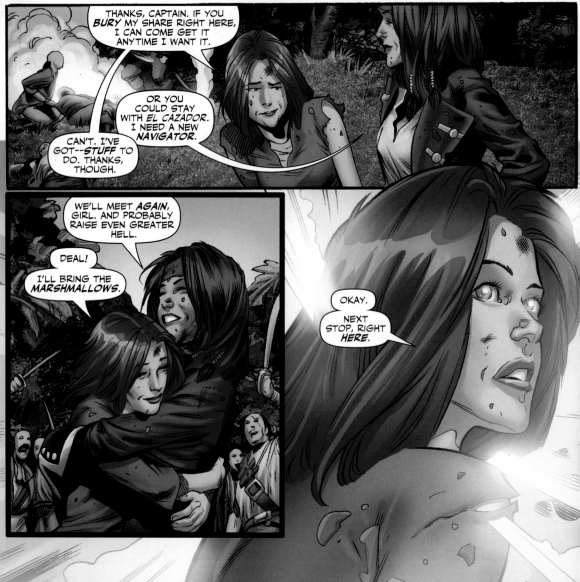

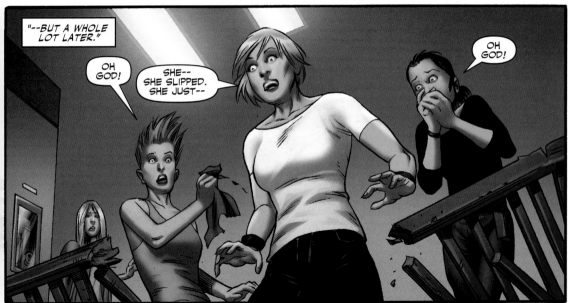

"--BUT A WHOLE LOT LATER."

OH GOD!

SHE-- SHE SLIPPED. SHE JUST--

OH GOD!

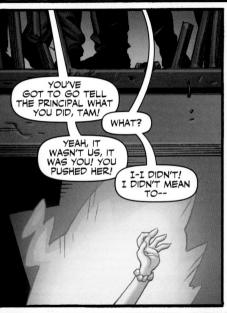

YOU'VE GOT TO GO TELL THE PRINCIPAL WHAT YOU DID, TAM!

WHAT?

YEAH, IT WASN'T US, IT WAS YOU! YOU PUSHED HER!

I-I DIDN'T! I DIDN'T MEAN TO--

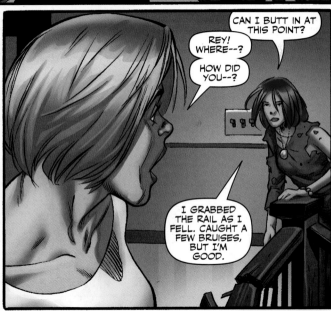

CAN I BUTT IN AT THIS POINT?

REY! WHERE--?

HOW DID YOU--?

I GRABBED THE RAIL AS I FELL. CAUGHT A FEW BRUISES, BUT I'M GOOD.

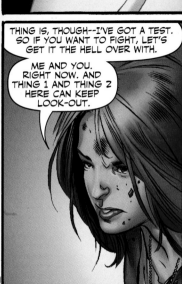

THING IS, THOUGH--I'VE GOT A TEST. SO IF YOU WANT TO FIGHT, LET'S GET IT THE HELL OVER WITH.

ME AND YOU. RIGHT NOW. AND THING 1 AND THING 2 HERE CAN KEEP LOOK-OUT.

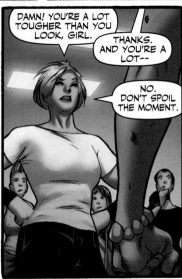

DAMN! YOU'RE A LOT TOUGHER THAN YOU LOOK, GIRL.

THANKS. AND YOU'RE A LOT--

NO. DON'T SPOIL THE MOMENT.

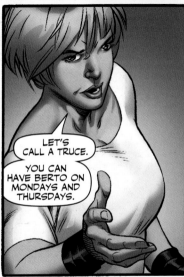

LET'S CALL A TRUCE.

YOU CAN HAVE BERTO ON MONDAYS AND THURSDAYS.

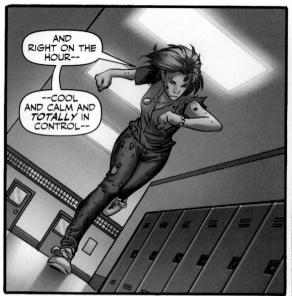

AND RIGHT ON THE HOUR--

--COOL AND CALM AND *TOTALLY* IN CONTROL--

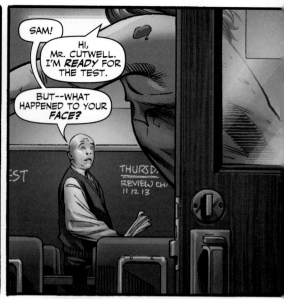

SAM!

HI, MR. CUTWELL. I'M *READY* FOR THE TEST.

BUT--WHAT HAPPENED TO YOUR *FACE?*

THURSD.
REVIEW CH.
11 12 13

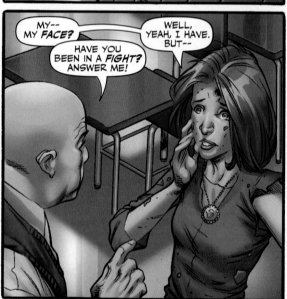

MY-- MY *FACE?*

WELL, YEAH, I HAVE. BUT--

HAVE YOU BEEN IN A *FIGHT?* ANSWER ME!

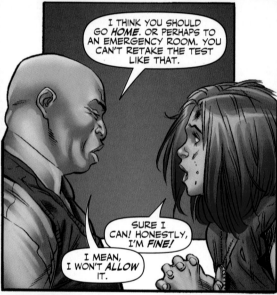

I THINK YOU SHOULD GO *HOME.* OR PERHAPS TO AN EMERGENCY ROOM. YOU CAN'T RETAKE THE TEST LIKE THAT.

SURE I CAN! HONESTLY, I'M *FINE!*

I MEAN, I WON'T *ALLOW* IT.

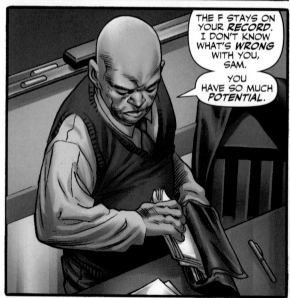

THE F STAYS ON YOUR *RECORD.* I DON'T KNOW WHAT'S *WRONG* WITH YOU, SAM.

YOU HAVE SO MUCH *POTENTIAL.*

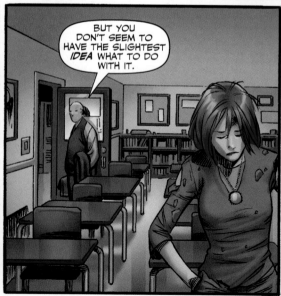

BUT YOU DON'T SEEM TO HAVE THE SLIGHTEST *IDEA* WHAT TO DO WITH IT.

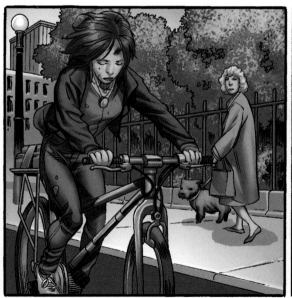

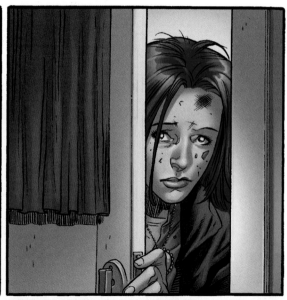

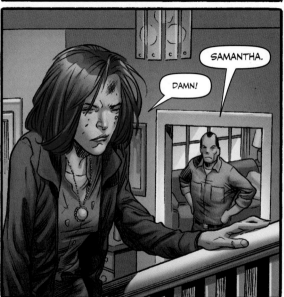

DAMN!

SAMANTHA.

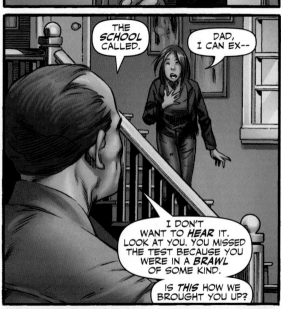

THE *SCHOOL* CALLED.

DAD, I CAN EX--

I DON'T WANT TO *HEAR* IT. LOOK AT YOU. YOU MISSED THE TEST BECAUSE YOU WERE IN A *BRAWL* OF SOME KIND.

IS *THIS* HOW WE BROUGHT YOU UP?

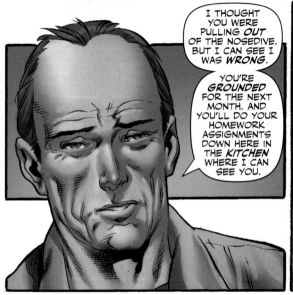

I THOUGHT YOU WERE PULLING *OUT* OF THE NOSEDIVE. BUT I CAN SEE I WAS *WRONG.*

YOU'RE *GROUNDED* FOR THE NEXT MONTH. AND YOU'LL DO YOUR HOMEWORK ASSIGNMENTS DOWN HERE IN THE *KITCHEN* WHERE I CAN SEE YOU.

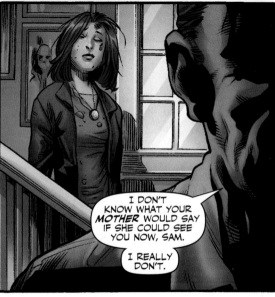

I DON'T KNOW WHAT YOUR *MOTHER* WOULD SAY IF SHE COULD SEE YOU NOW, SAM.

I REALLY DON'T.

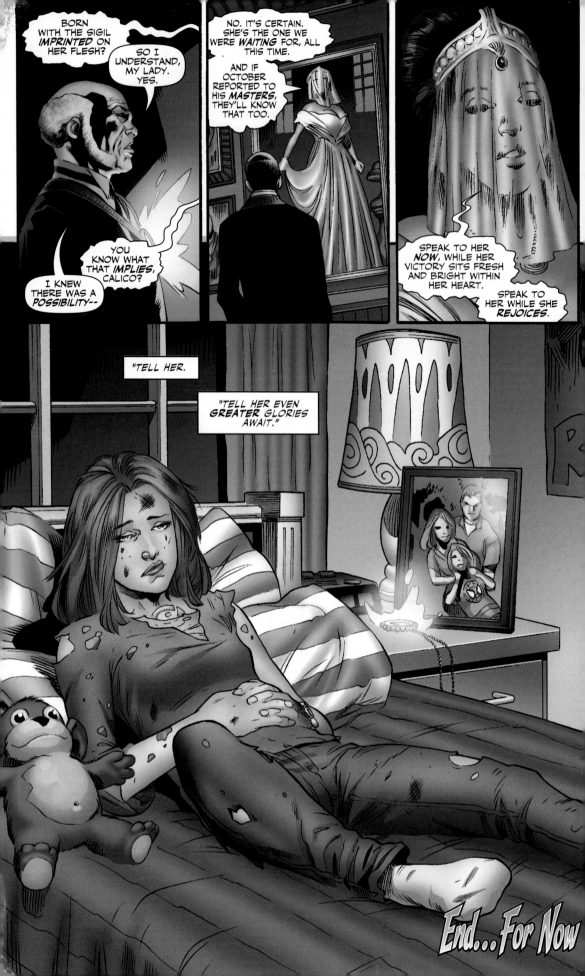

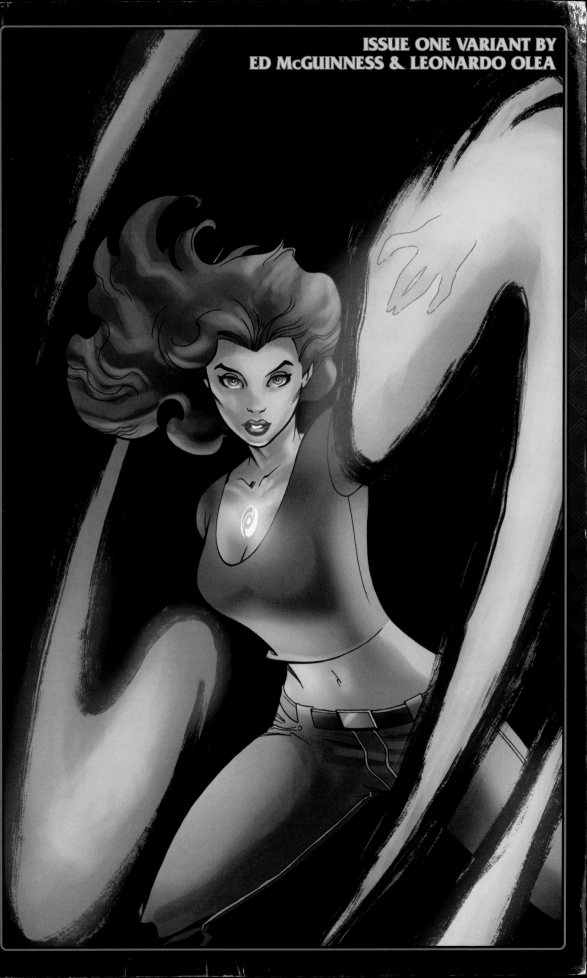
ISSUE ONE VARIANT BY
ED McGUINNESS & LEONARDO OLEA

CHARACTER DESIGNS
BY LEONARD KIRK

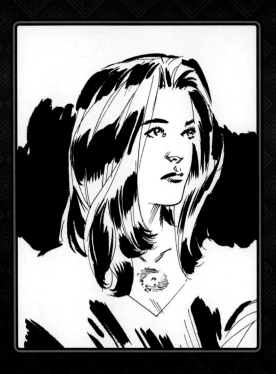

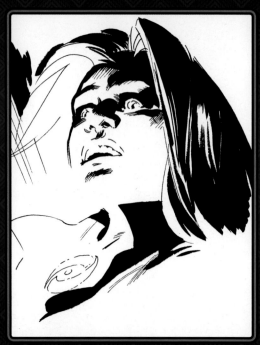

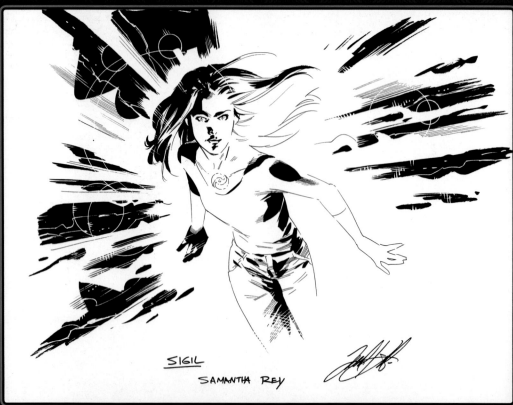

SIGIL
SAMANTHA REY

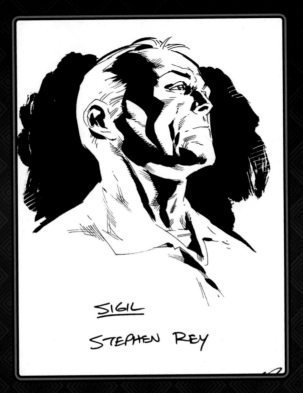

SIGIL

STEPHEN REY

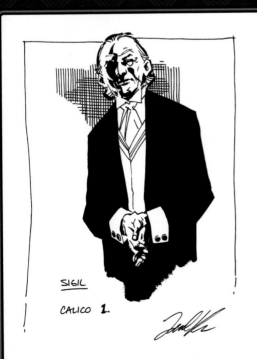

SIGIL

CALICO 1.

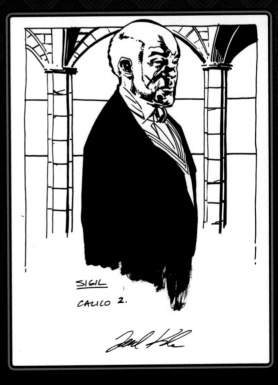

SIGIL

CALICO 2.

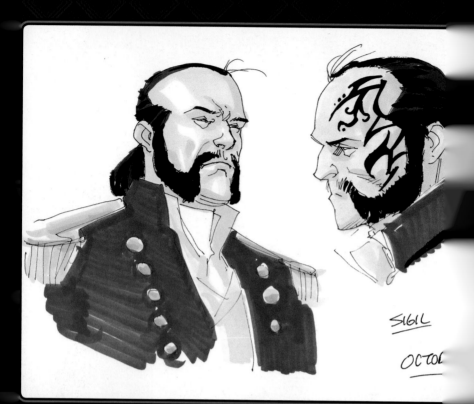

SIGIL

OCTOB

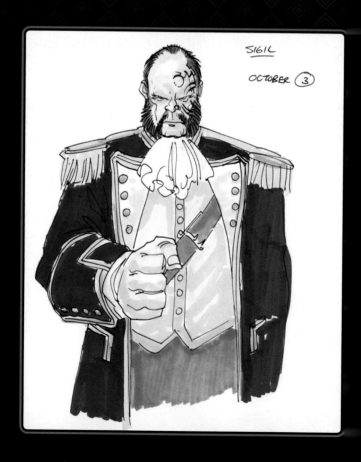

SIGIL

OCTOBER ③

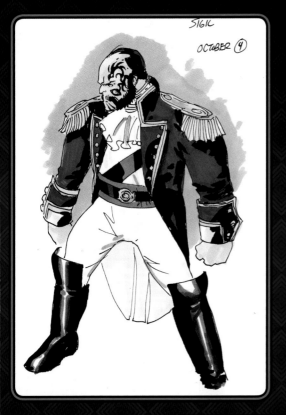

SIGIL

OCTOBER 4

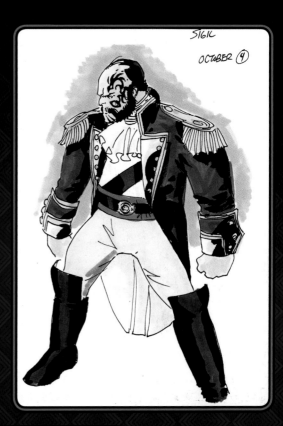

SIGIL

OCTOBER 4

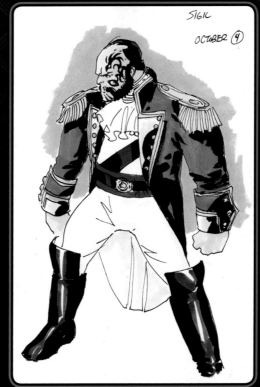

SIGIL

OCTOBER 4

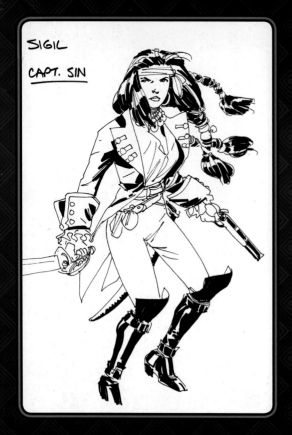

SIGIL

CAPT. SIN

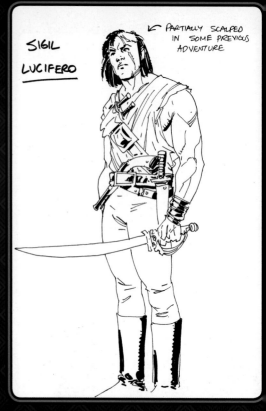

SIGIL

LUCIFERO

PARTIALLY SCALPED
IN SOME PREVIOUS
ADVENTURE

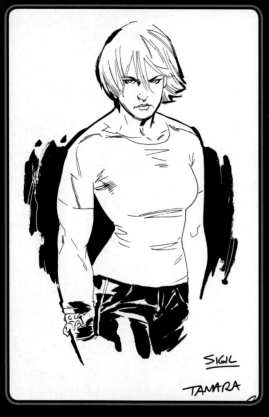

SIGIL

TAMARA

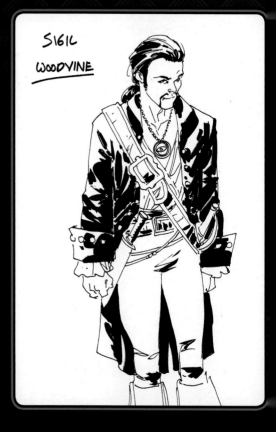

SIGIL

WOODVINE

NAVIGATING
THE ADVENTURE
WITH
MIKE CAREY

MARVEL: Sigil is an epoch-spanning, fantasy epic of the tallest order. How do you manage to anchor the story with Samantha Rey? How is she a relatable character in this fantasy setting?

MIKE CAREY: I think in any fantasy, it's the real world stuff that's the anchor. If you make the reader believe in and invest in that, then the fantasy has weight and momentum when it comes in. I made Sam my starting point when I was planning the story. I gave a lot of thought to her family life, the school and social context – the small observational details that hopefully make her seem like a real teenaged girl. It helps that I have a teenaged daughter myself: I stole a lot of Louise to animate Sam. Having said that, we meet Sam in a somewhat extreme situation. She's recently bereaved, still struggling to cope, and off her stride in a number of important ways. Paradoxically, I think that helps us to get to know her better quite quickly.

MARVEL: We think it's safe to say that Sigil draws on a cast culled from radically different time periods, alien worlds, and planes of reality. What are just some of the locales readers can expect to visit during the course of the series?

MC: In this opening story arc, we've limited ourselves to three sets of locations. We've got scenes set in the present day, scenes set in and around California in the late seventeenth or early eighteenth century – the time of the buccaneers, essentially – and then a third setting which is totally outside normal time and space. We wanted to establish what the sigils can do and some of the parameters for how they work, and we thought the best way to do that was by making sure that all the settings here are very fully realized. Of course, both in the present and in the past, we won't necessarily be meeting people who belong only in those particular times and places...

MARVEL: As mentioned, Sigil takes place on a huge canvas, incorporating elements of several different genres. At its core, what makes CrossGen a different animal than the mainstream Marvel Universe?

MC: That's a big question. At least part of the answer is the mix of genres, which you've already referred to. The MU is accommodating to a wide range of genres – horror, Western, romance, comedy, and so on – but its beating heart is the super hero genre, which – although it has its origins in sci-fi – is a complete and self-defining thing. The heart of the CrossGen Universe, arguably, is fantasy – costumed heroes can be found there, but they're not where its center of gravity lies. It's a broad, fantasy cosmos based on a small number of tropes that play very effectively off each other, and of course the sigil is one of those tropes. That makes for a different approach to storytelling and to character creation. Some of the best CrossGen books had big core casts and were built on a premise rather than a character. Most super hero books put the character, or a small group of characters, firmly at the center.

MARVEL: You've made a career out of creating some really unique, resonant characters – Samantha Rey seems like one of those. What makes her stand out from so many other female protagonists in popular fiction?

MC: I like Sam because she's got a mixture of vulnerability and strength. When we first meet her, she's been through a lot and she's feeling pretty fragile – but when she's thrown into the midst of this chaos and conflict, she discovers sides of her own nature that she didn't know were there. In some ways, she's a classic underdog who gets a chance to make good. But she's also a girl with a hugely passionate and warm-hearted nature, who never really feels entirely comfortable in the role of a soldier – which in some ways is what she's being pushed towards. Those tensions make her a lot of fun to write.

MARVEL: What is your favorite thing about working with characters in the CrossGen Universe as opposed to traditional super hero stories?

MC: I guess sci-fi and heroic fantasy are areas that I haven't worked in all that often. They're the axletree of the CrossGen Universe, and they encourage you to come at things from odd angles. From the start, we were thinking about how to move away from the good versus evil staples of traditional fantasy and create a cosmic struggle that was based on a different set of oppositions – although, to begin with, it might seem like we're setting ourselves firmly in that tradition. It's a question of referencing ground that seems familiar, and then pulling it out from under the reader in interesting and unexpected ways. Of course, that's also what a lot of my favorite super hero stories do...

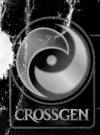

TALKING CROSSGEN
WITH DAVID GABRIEL, S.V.P. OF PUBLISHING SALES

MARVEL: What does Marvel hope to achieve with the CrossGen properties?

DAVID GABRIEL: We're looking to expand our universes a bit and add some fresh new genres to our mix. There are some great concepts that exist within the older CrossGen universe of characters and this is a great opportunity to reimagine these characters and stories with a Marvel sensibility.

MARVEL: What made Marvel decide to launch the CrossGen imprint with Sigil & Ruse?

DG: Honestly this was an editorial and creative decision. We cast the net wide to see what kinds of pitches we could get back using all the characters and titles that exist within this new universe and bringing in a range of new ideas from our extended creative pool. We had narrowed it down to five, and we thought that Sigil made the most sense to launch with because of its original importance to the CrossGen universe. And combining Mark Waid and Ruse seemed like a surefire win!

MARVEL: What future plans does Marvel have for CrossGen and what other titles will we see?

DG: We have a plan for which books we are going to release and when but we don't want to tip our hand just yet. There are a lot of titles to choose from so we're really taking our time and working on these books to make them the best possible stories we can.

MARVEL: Super hero stories are Marvel's bread and butter. What are fans going to be attracted to about the CrossGen properties and how does Marvel plan to make these non-super hero tales viable?

DG: I think a few years back we proved that Marvel isn't just about super hero stories anymore with books like Dark Tower, Halo, Wizard of Oz, Pride and Prejudice, Ender's Game, and even Zombies and now we see the CrossGen properties as another extension of our reaching out into new genres of mystery, fantasy, sci-fi, horror, sword and sorcery, and a whole slew of other untapped universes for us.

We'll be taking the same sensibilities that we use in our super hero storytelling and using those within this new universe. We'll be using the best talent Marvel has to offer to create stunning tales of these imaginative worlds. We'll be getting to the core elements that made

these stories resonate with so many fans years ago and reignite those passions for these stories. I think we'll be finding the "super hero" in these concepts and really making them Marvel!

MARVEL: Does Marvel have any plans to reprint the old CrossGen material?

DG: Not at present. We've talked about it, perhaps launching some digitally later on. But in looking at everything we want to accomplish, we really want these new series to be seen as fresh new concepts. They're not continuations of the originals so we want to avoid any confusion. No one will need to read the old stories to know what's going on or who these characters and titles are. This is a brand new universe for Marvel to explore and reinvigorate. In a way it's like looking at the Ultimate Universe and trying to match those up with the Marvel U masterworks of similar titles. We may do it down the road for nostalgia, but for now, we want to let these new books stand on their own.

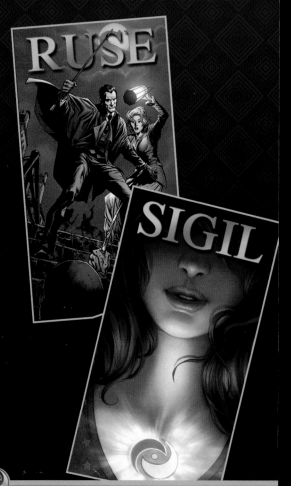